Overcoming
Allergies

Dr Christina Scott-Moncrieff
MB ChB MFHom

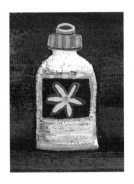

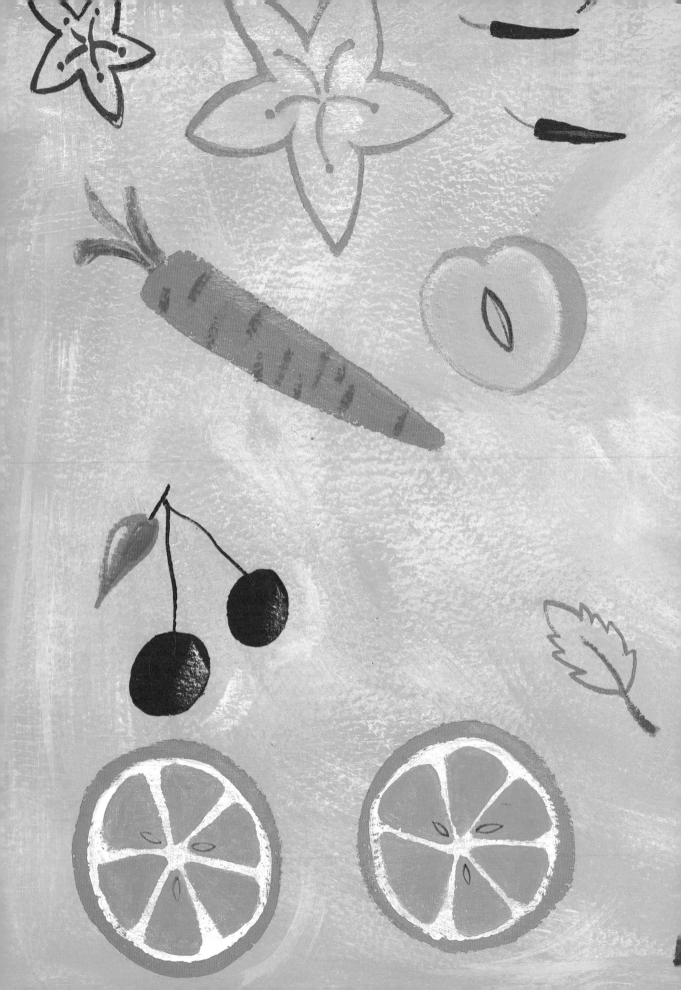

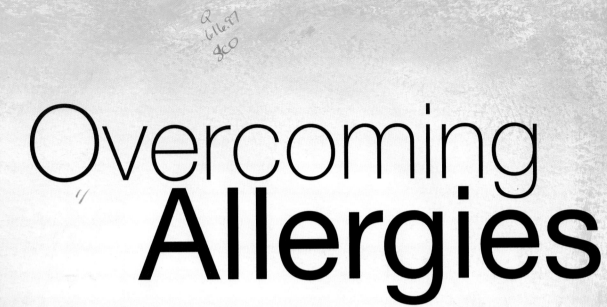

Overcoming
Allergies

Dr Christina Scott-Moncrieff

MB ChB MFHom

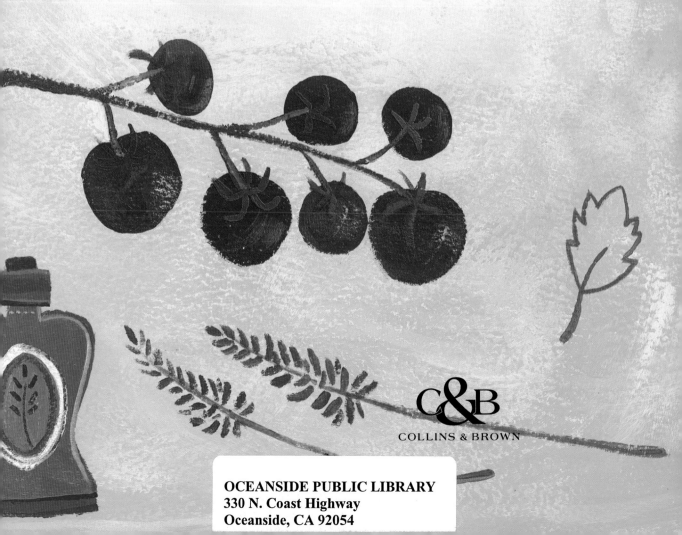

C&B

COLLINS & BROWN

The author and publishers would like to thank Michelle Berriedale-Johnson for the delicious recipes featured in this book.

First published in Great Britain in 2002
by Collins & Brown Limited
64 Brewery Road
London N7 9NT

A member of the Chrysalis Group plc

1 3 5 7 9 8 6 4 2

British Library Cataloguing-in-Publication Data:
A catalogue record for this book is available from the British Library.

ISBN 1 85585 914 9

Commissioned by Grace Cheetham
Project managed by Emma Baxter
Art direction by Anne-Marie Bulat
Designed by Emily Cook
Edited by Judith Hannam
Illustrations by Tiffany Lynch/New Division
Recipes by Michelle Berriedale-Johnson

Reproduction by Classicscan, Singapore
Printed and bound in Singapore by Craftprint

The diets and the information in this book are for information only and are not intended to replace appropriate advice from a qualified practitioner. Always consult your health practitioner before adopting any suggestions in this book.

Contents

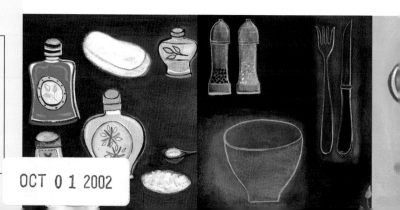

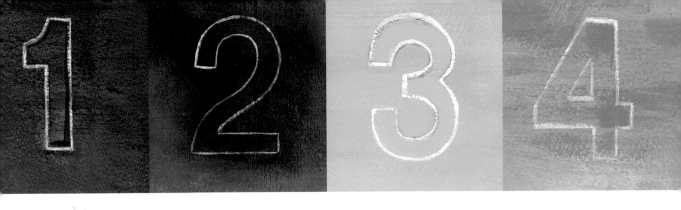

Introduction

More and more people are suffering from allergies. Estimates suggest that one in three of us in the West will suffer from an allergy at some point during our lives, and conditions such as asthma, and anaphylatic reactions to foods such as peanuts, are becoming increasingly common. Conventional treatments should not be lightly dismissed, as they can be lifesavers, but all too often they merely suppress symptoms rather than provide a cure, and many have adverse side effects.

The aim of this book is to let you take charge of your allergies. The main focus is on the comprehensive diet plan, but it also lists the many complementary therapies and natural remedies that can help you combat the underlying causes of your allergies and to achieve full health and wellbeing.

The first step is to identify your allergy and its cause, as well as any other non-allergic triggers or aggravating factors, so that these can be avoided as far as possible. The second step involves improving your general health – by eating a good diet, reducing the stress in your life and minimizing your exposure to chemicals that need to be changed into safer compounds before being excreted from your body. Coping with stress and foreign chemicals uses up a surprising amount of energy – which could be better directed towards enjoying life! If your allergic symptoms persist after following the suggested self-help measures, you may need to consider consulting a therapist who specializes in alternative and complementary therapies.

USING THIS BOOK

Part 1 describes the most common allergic conditions. For each condition, self-help measures are given, together with references directing you to the pages where you can obtain more information. Dietary changes are suggested for a number of allergies, and you will be directed either to follow the Diet Plan in **Part 2**, or to consider other dietary changes that may be helpful. The Diet Plan includes a structured approach to identifying foods that may be causing symptoms, and advice on how to return to a more normal way of eating.

You will find a number of conditions mentioned in **Part 1** – such as irritable bowel syndrome (IBS) and arthritis – that are often not treated as allergies by conventional doctors. Those who specialize in environmental medicine, however, frequently find that the symptoms caused by these conditions can be improved by treating them in much the same way as allergies, and for this reason they are included here. You will also find sections on chronic tiredness and Candida, both of which are often associated with the tendency to develop allergies. Such allergies usually disappear when the tiredness and Candida are treated.

Combating your allergy by adopting a healthy lifestyle is covered in **Part 3**. This section looks at choosing a healthy diet, introducing regular exercise and managing your stress levels. For allergy sufferers, creating a lo-allergy environment is important, and there is advice on how to do this both at home and work, and in your garden.

Part 4 deals with obtaining professional help from either your doctor or from practitioners of a wide range of alternative and complementary therapies, including traditional Chinese and Indian medical systems, naturopathy, homeopathy, massage, aromatherapy, osteopathy, shiatsu, hydrotherapy, hypnotherapy, healing, autogenic training and biofeedback.

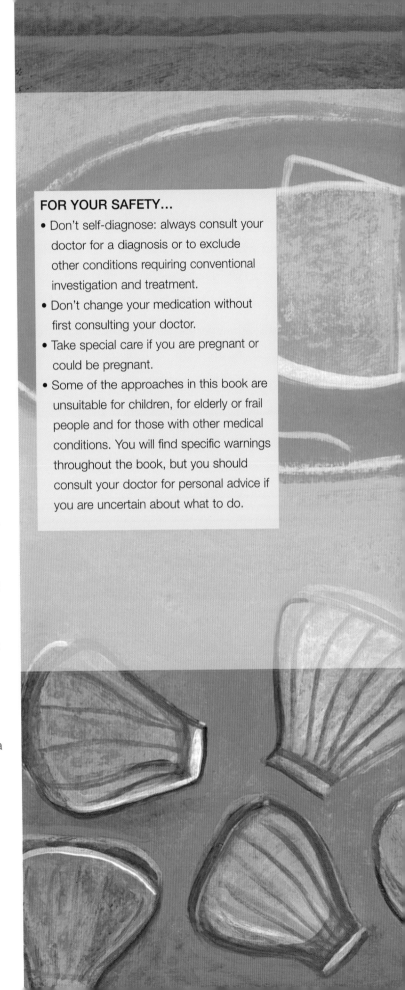

FOR YOUR SAFETY...

- Don't self-diagnose: always consult your doctor for a diagnosis or to exclude other conditions requiring conventional investigation and treatment.
- Don't change your medication without first consulting your doctor.
- Take special care if you are pregnant or could be pregnant.
- Some of the approaches in this book are unsuitable for children, for elderly or frail people and for those with other medical conditions. You will find specific warnings throughout the book, but you should consult your doctor for personal advice if you are uncertain about what to do.

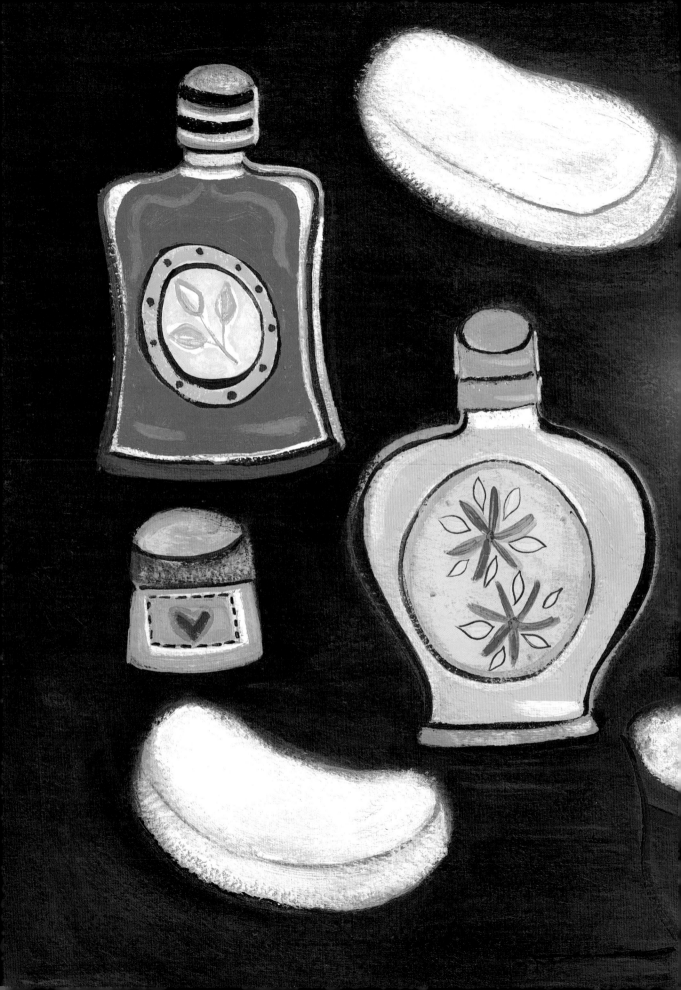

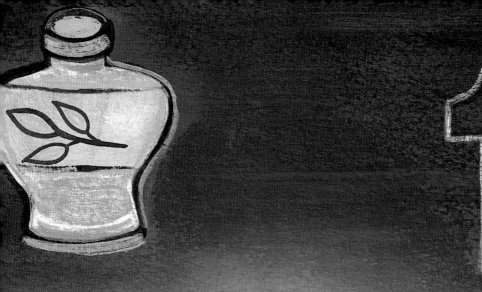

1

Taking
charge

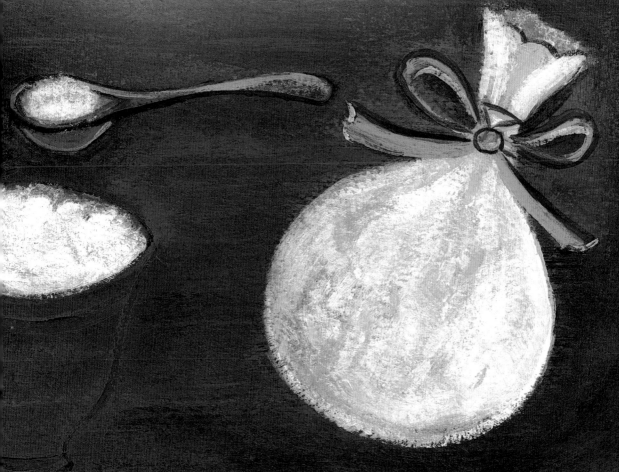

What is an allergy?

An allergy is an adverse reaction involving the immune system, which follows contact with a substance that is normally harmless.

In many types of allergy the symptoms occur very rapidly and usually involve the part of the body that has been in contact with the 'harmless' substance. Most allergic reactions occur in the mouth, nose, lungs, digestive tract, or on the skin. So in hay fever, for example, contact with grass pollen causes the nose and eyes to discharge, frequent sneezing, and the eyes, nose, roof of the mouth and even the ears to feel itchy.

The symptoms occur when the immune system, for reasons we do not understand, over-reacts to a substance from which it believes the body needs protection. Such substances are known as allergens, and they can trigger an allergic reaction when they come in contact with the body – by being touched, inhaled, eaten or injected.

Confusion can sometimes arise because symptoms that are similar or even identical to those produced by an allergic reaction can occur without the immune system apparently being involved. For example, frequent sneezing and a runny nose are allergic reactions when they are caused by exposure to grass pollen, but not when they result from chemical irritation, such as when chopping onions, or from a common cold.

REACTIONS TO CHEMICALS

Some people appear to be sensitive to chemicals that enter the body either through the skin or by

NON-ALLERGIC FOOD REACTIONS

Certain foods can produce symptoms similar to those triggered by an allergy or food intolerance, but the cause is entirely different. Non-allergic food reactions can be difficult to treat, but your doctor will be able to help. Examples include:

- Symptoms caused by foods that contain or release **histamine** (see p.73), which is one of the chemicals released by the immune system in an allergic reaction.
- Symptoms triggered by foods containing **chemicals** that act in much the same way as a drug, e.g. caffeine (see p.73).

- Symptoms caused by the body's inability to produce certain digestive secretions. For example, most people of African and Asian descent are unable, after infancy, to digest the sugar in milk; other people cannot break down all the proteins in wheat, milk or corn (maize).
- Toxic symptoms triggered by certain foods, such as red kidney beans, that have not been cooked correctly.
- Symptoms of food poisoning caused by eating contaminated food.

being inhaled. If you are sensitive to chemicals –
such as fumes from petrol or paint, perfumes,
pesticides and cigarette smoke – you may
experience a number of symptoms, including
migraines, fatigue, abdominal pain, rhinitis,
eczema and urticaria when you come into contact
with them. (See also **chemical sensitivity**, p.48.)

REACTIONS TO FOOD

Many people experience various adverse
reactions to food, in fact one person in six has a
food allergy, which can range from relatively mild
to very severe. Usually, it is a lifelong condition,
which recurs whenever the culprit food is eaten,
so avoiding it is essential. Any food can be
involved, but the commonest culprits are peanuts
(groundnuts), fish, shellfish, papaya and
strawberries. The trouble begins when the food
comes into contact with the mouth, causing
tingling and local swelling. Other symptoms
include nausea, sickness and stomach cramps.
An **urticarial rash** (see p.20), **wheezing** (see
p.30) and coughing may also occur. In rare cases
anaphylaxis may develop (see p.13).

WHAT IS FOOD INTOLERANCE?

In food intolerance, the immune system does not
appear to be involved. In addition, the symptoms
– which include **headaches** (see p.40), **tiredness**
(see p.42), depression, painful or aching muscles,
mouth ulcers (see p.23), digestive disorders,
such as **irritable bowel syndrome** (see p.34),
and **arthritis** (see p.46) – are usually less
immediate and more likely to involve distant parts
of the body, such as the brain. Any food can
cause intolerance, but the commonest culprits are
those eaten frequently, such as wheat, eggs and
milk. It is best to avoid the culprit foods, but unlike
food allergy, you can reintroduce them eventually.

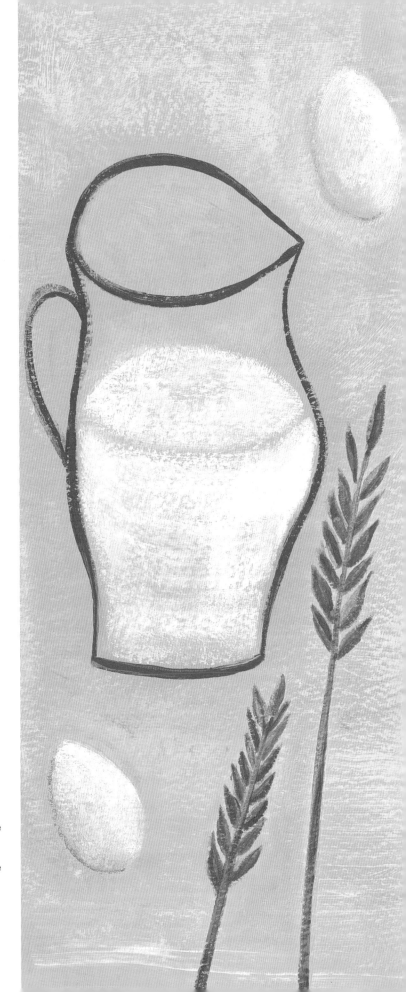

What causes allergies?

Allergies are thought to result from a combination of inherited susceptibility and adverse environmental conditions. The way in which the tendency is inherited is complex and not fully understood. Even more puzzling is why some members of a family develop an allergy while others do not. Identical twins, for example, have exactly the same genes, and may also have similar positive RAST tests (see p.137), yet in some cases only one of them will develop allergic symptoms.

The environment in which we live and work can play a significant part. For example, the risk of developing an allergy is known to be increased in people exposed to allergens in the first few weeks of life (see p.131). Infections, such as flu, can also trigger the start of an allergy, especially if, at the same time, the person has suffered an emotional trauma, such as bereavement.

Diet is another factor. People with allergic conditions are often deficient in minerals, especially magnesium (see p.113), although it is not clear whether this deficit is a cause of allergy, or its result. Recent research has also indicated that eating fresh fruit and vegetables provides children with some protection from developing asthma.

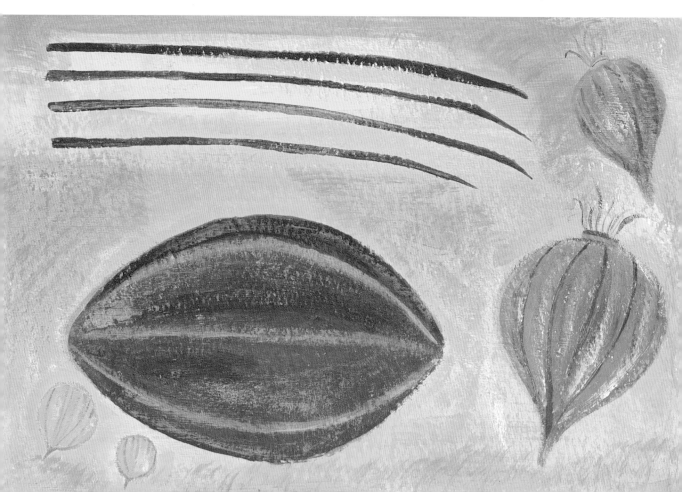

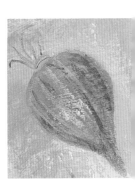

ANAPHYLAXIS

Anaphylaxis, or anaphylactic shock, is a severe allergic reaction involving the whole body, which can come on very quickly after contact with the allergen responsible, such as a sting or a particular food. Fortunately, it is rare. The symptoms include:

- Itching and swelling around the face, inside the mouth, including the tongue, and the throat. As a result breathing may be difficult and wheezing may start.
- The skin may become flushed and an **urticarial rash** can develop (see p.20).
- A very rapid heartbeat; yet at the same time there may be a feeling of weakness, because blood pressure often drops.
- Stomach cramps and nausea.
- Collapse and loss of consciousness may follow.

Urgent first aid is needed. If the victim has had a previous attack and carries adrenaline and antihistamine medicine, these should be administered quickly. The adrenaline is either injected or, if prescribed as an inhaler, sprayed inside the cheek in some cases both may be required. (Caution: avoid giving adrenaline to anyone with a heart condition, unless it has been prescribed specifically for that person.) Always send either for medical help or an ambulance. Even if recovery seems to occur, professional advice should still be obtained, as a relapse may follow when the effect of the medication wears off.

While waiting, loosen clothing at the neck and waist, and assist the victim to lie down, as this helps to raise their blood pressure, especially if you can also raise their legs and feet a little. If swelling around the neck and throat is making breathing difficult, you can raise the upper part of the body on pillows or cushions, but keep the head bent gently backwards to keep the airway open. If the cause was a sting from a bee, any remaining sting should be removed (see p.15). If the victim starts to vomit, turn the head to one side.

SENSIBLE PRECAUTIONS

The first attack of anaphylaxis may come out of the blue, but in many cases there will have been a previous reaction to a sting or item of food. If you suffer from any reaction it is certainly worth consulting your doctor, because reactions tend to become more severe each time they occur. Your doctor may be able to arrange for **desensitization** (see p.137), or may prescribe medication.

If you have had a previous anaphylactic reaction, it is important to carry your medication with you at all times. Adrenaline is only effective for a certain period, so make a note of the expiry date in your diary or on a calendar, to remind yourself when you need to obtain a further supply. It may also be sensible to wear a bracelet or pendant inscribed with the details of your allergy.

Pets and pests can cause allergies

If allergies run in your family, the chances are high that you will also become allergic to the other, non-human occupants of your house, such as pets and pests.

Although cats are very clean animals, they are more likely to cause allergic reactions than dogs because the protein in their saliva, released as they lick themselves, becomes airborne as it dries. This protein is extremely persistent and can still be found in houses years after the cats have left. Cats, dogs, horses and other furry animals can also cause allergic symptoms from the dander, which is a form of dandruff, in their fur. The fur often also carries other allergens, such as **pollens** (see p.27, p.28). People who keep birds can become allergic to their feathers; others can react to feathers in pillows and soft furnishings. Allergies have also been reported to particles of skin shed by cockroaches.

Faeces and droppings are common sources of allergens, the house-dust mite being a frequent culprit in temperate countries (see p.19). Allergens also occur in dog faeces and urine, cockroach faeces and bird droppings.

INSECT STINGS

Insects protect themselves by their ability to sting and inject a small amount of poisonous venom into their victims. For most people this injected toxin is a passing irritation, but other people can have an allergic reaction, which may be severe, especially if they have been stung repeatedly by the same type of insect.

In general, honeybees and bumblebees only sting when severely provoked, but they leave their sting behind, attached to a sac, which

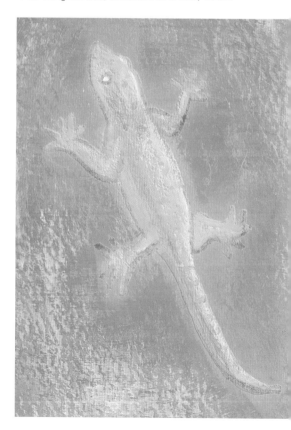

Reptiles are probably the safest pets for the allergic family!

continues to inject venom. The sting should be removed as quickly as possible, either by flicking it off with a fingernail, or with tweezers applied as near to the skin as possible, to avoid squeezing the venom sac. Wasps and hornets tend to be more aggressive, but do not leave their stings behind. They are often drawn to sources of sugar, so can arrive at a picnic or hide in fruit on a tree. It is best to avoid sudden movements when they approach; instead just walk quietly away.

AFTER YOU ARE STUNG

For stings in or near the mouth, or stings that swell rapidly, always obtain medical advice (see also **anaphylaxis,** p.13) as well as applying first aid treatemnt.

- **Take an antihistamine** to relieve irritation and paracetamol (acetominophen), if needed, for pain. Useful homeopathic medicines for bee and wasp stings include Apis mellifica 6c, one tablet every 15 minutes for an hour or so; and Ledum 6c, one tablet every 15 minutes for four doses, then one tablet every three hours until the pain subsides (for infants and children use 6–10 granules). For further information see p.116.
- **Apply an ice pack** for a maximum of 10 minutes. Alternatively, for bee stings, apply a paste made up of water and bicarbonate of soda (baking soda). For wasp stings, apply a cotton wool pad soaked in vinegar.

AVOIDING INSECT STINGS

- **Cover up well**, and do not walk about barefoot out of doors. Avoid brightly coloured clothes, especially floral prints.
- **Wear gloves and a hat** when gardening, and gloves (and a helmet) when riding a bicycle or motorbike.
- **Avoid perfumes**, including scented deodorants, sunscreens and cosmetics, as these products will attract insects. Sweat and the carbon dioxide in exhaled breath also attracts them, so take special care when exercising outside.
- **Take precautions when cooking or eating** outside, or when picking fruit, particularly apples, plums and pears. Keep food covered and avoid places where animals are fed. Inspect food and liquids for insects as you eat, and never drink directly from a can.
- **Prevent insects entering your house** by keeping your doors and windows shut, or, if you prefer, covered with a fine netting. Also keep any food covered.

REACTING TO STINGS AND BITES

If you have had **urticaria** (see p.20) or other symptoms – such as swelling around the face, wheezing, nausea or diarrhoea – after an insect sting or bite, consult your doctor. Reactions tend to become worse each time they occur.

Eczema

Atopic eczema is a condition that usually starts in infancy and often clears up during childhood, but may persist into adult life. The word atopic suggests that the condition is the result of an inherited tendency to develop allergies, and close relatives often have eczema, asthma or other allergic conditions. The term eczema simply means dry, inflamed skin, which is normally itchy.

Most adults try not to scratch affected areas, but frequently do so in their sleep, which makes the skin weep, causing it to become infected. As the skin heals, it becomes itchy again and the scratching often restarts. This cycle of scratching and healing leaves the skin thickened; there may also be changes in the pigmentation, resulting in patches of unusually dark or pale skin. Although eczema usually starts in infancy it can occasionally surface in adult life. However, many children with eczema become free of it by the time they are adults, even though their skin often remains dry and they may be prone to **contact allergic dermatitis** (see p.24).

CAUSE

Unfortunately, we do not know the cause of eczema, which can come and go for no obvious reason. Recent research suggests that in some people eczema may be linked with either a lack of **essential fatty acids** in the diet (see p.110) or a reduced ability to process them (see box).

CAUTION

No child with eczema should be put on a mini-elimination diet to test for food intolerance, unless they are under the direct supervision of a doctor experienced in this approach. Children with eczema often grow rather slowly and it is important that they do not become malnourished. In addition, some children, especially boys, have, on rare occasions, reacted severely when foods have been reintroduced and, for this reason, doctors often advise that testing be done in hospital.

ESSENTIAL FATTY ACIDS

Nutritionists class certain oils as 'essential', which means that they cannot be made in the body, but have to be obtained from the diet. Deficiency in these oils, chemically known as essential fatty acids (or EFAs), can cause dryness and inflammation of the skin, as a healthy skin needs plenty of oil to remain supple and waterproof. Even when the diet is adequate, some people with eczema appear to have a deficiency in the way they process one of these essential oils, known as gamma-linoleic acid (GLA). Evening primrose seeds are a rich source of this oil, and evening primrose oil supplements have been found to reverse this deficiency in some people, when taken regularly, but you will probably need to continue for a few weeks before you see an improvement.

WHAT YOU CAN DO

1 **Keep the skin well moisturized and cool** to reduce itching and minimize the risk of infection (see **home remedies** on p.20). Preparations rich in essential fats (see opposite) can also help, but they have a short shelf-life, as the oils soon become rancid. When necessary, use low-strength steroid creams to contain the symptoms.

p.20

2 Avoid **skin irritants** (see **home remedies** on p.18). You can become sensitive to the constituents of almost any cream or ointment, so stop using those that appear to be aggravating your skin. Your pharmacist will be able to recommend alternatives.

p.18

3 Ask your doctor to arrange skin or blood tests to confirm or exclude allergy to house-dust mites, pollens or pets. Allergy to these can occur when they come into contact with skin that has already been damaged by eczema. If the tests are positive, take appropriate avoidance measures (see p.136 for **allergy testing**, p.19 for **house-dust mites**, p.27, p.28 for **pollens**, p.14 for **pets**, p.137 for **desensitization**).

Parts 1 & 4

4 For a few weeks, avoid foods that contain or release histamine, as you may have a **false food allergy** (see p.73). If your skin improves, you may find that not eating them when the skin is particularly inflamed brings some relief.

p.73

5 Adolescents and adults should consider the possibility that they have **contact allergic dermatitis** (see p.24) rather than eczema.

p.24

6 Make sure you eat a healthy diet containing an adequate supply of **essential fatty acids** (see p.110) and consider taking an evening primrose oil supplement for a few weeks to see if your skin improves. For dosage, follow the manufacturer's advice.

p.110

7 Consider the possibility of food intolerance. The extent to which foods cause eczema is unknown, but there are undoubtedly some people whose eczema responds dramatically when the foods to which they are intolerant are removed from their diet. If you wish to try this approach, start the **mini-elimination diet** (see p.58).

p.58

8 Helpful alternative therapies include **stress management** (see p.122), **aromatherapy** (see p.150) and **hypnotherapy** (p.151). **Homeopathy** can sometimes be very helpful, but it can also make eczema much worse, so you should always consult a homeopathic practitioner, preferably one who is also a doctor (see p.146).

Parts 3 & 4

HOME REMEDIES

Certain substances can irritate the skin without being allergens and, for many people with eczema, avoiding these substances can effectively reduce inflammation. There are simple measures you can take to protect your skin and these include:

- **Using emollients** (such as aqueous cream) instead of soap; your doctor or pharmacist will advise you if you are uncertain about which product to use.
- **Installing a water softener** if you live in a hard water area and your eczema clears when you visit a soft water area.
- **Taking brief baths** (15 minutes maximum) in warm (not hot) water, using an emollient – such as an aqueous cream or a handful of oatmeal placed in a sock and tied under the hot tap so that the water runs through it as it fills the tub. Then wrap yourself in a dry towel without rubbing, and apply aqueous cream or other emollient immediately afterwards, even if the skin is not completely dry.
- **Wearing pure cotton clothing** next to the skin, as wool and artificial fibres can irritate. Clothes, towels and bedding should all be washed in non-irritant soap or non-biological washing powder.
- **Keeping fingernails short** and clean will help to reduce damage to the skin and prevent the introduction of infection if you tend to scratch at night.
- **Staying cool** (see p.20).
- **Avoiding smoking** and smoky places.

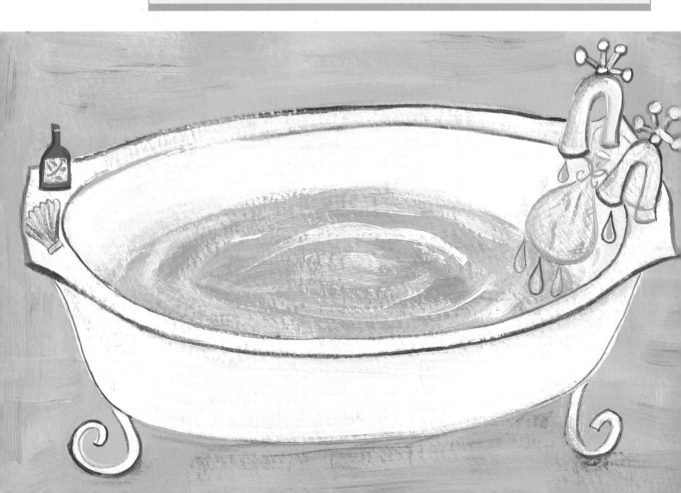

Dealing with the house-dust mite

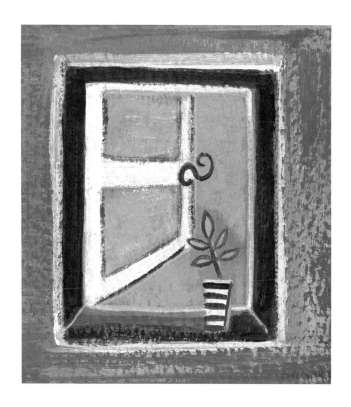

The faeces of house-dust mites cause several types of allergy (such as eczema, asthma, and rhinitis). The mites themselves eat discarded human skin scales and lurk in warm, damp places, such as in soft furnishings. Reducing their numbers sufficiently to avoid allergies requires considerable effort, so it's best to make sure that they are indeed responsible for your symptoms first, by asking your doctor to arrange the appropriate allergy tests.

To get rid of house-dust mites try the measures outlined below. It is often best to start in your bedroom as this is the place you spend several hours in each night:

- **Reduce damp** by ventilating your house well and sleeping with your window open (see also p.27). These measures may be as effective as getting rid of your carpets (see below).
- **Air bedding** every day in front of an open window or hang blankets and duvets on a washing line, especially on cold, crisp winter days. Use mite-proof coverings for mattresses and pillows.
- **Choose bedding that can be washed** at a high temperature 55–60°C (130–140°F), and wash it regularly to prevent build-up of skin flakes. Affected children who sleep in bunk beds should always occupy the top bunk.
- **Vacuum frequently**, using either a vacuum cleaner with a fine filter or one that passes the exhaust through water.
- **Avoid upholstered furniture**, replace curtains with blinds, and carpets with smooth floor coverings, such as cork, linoleum or vinyl. For comfort, use short-pile cotton mats that can be washed frequently at a high temperature.
- **Dust using a damp cloth**, rinse it under a tap and dry outside. Avoid clutter, which traps dust. Once a week, freeze soft toys overnight, and, if possible, wash them in hot water.
- **Affected infants who are still crawling should wear protective cotton clothing** that can be washed frequently.
- **Steam cleaning** kills dust mites very effectively. Proprietary sprays against the house-dust mite are available, but they don't always work very effectively, and they can also cause reactions in some people.

19

Urticaria or hives

The word urticaria literally means nettle rash, an appropriate description since the changes in the skin are usually similar to the itchy red bumps that form after a nettle sting. However, with urticaria much larger, raised red areas of skin can also occur.

Urticaria is a very itchy complaint, and if you develop the larger, raised areas it can also be quite painful. When urticaria occurs only around the mouth and throat, it is often in response to food and can make breathing difficult. In these cases it may be referred to as angioedema.

HOME REMEDIES

If you develop urticaria it is important to try and keep your skin cool in order to reduce itchiness. Try some of the following suggestions to ease your symptoms:

- **Staying out of the sun** and avoiding rooms that are too hot.
- **Wearing cotton clothes** and using cotton sheets on your bed next to your skin.
- **Applying ice cubes**, or ice wrapped in wet cotton material, to the affected area, for 5–10 minutes (no longer, to avoid frostbite), then using calamine lotion or a dressing of zinc oxide paste (available from a pharmacy).
- **Taking a cool, soothing bath**, and add a few drops of an oil that doesn't cause your skin to react, or instead some oatmeal, baking powder or cornflour (cornstarch). Avoid soap. Wrap yourself in a towel, but do not rub yourself with it, and then apply aqueous cream or an other perfume-free moisturizer, even if your skin is not completely dry.

- **Homeopaths** use a number of medicines, including Apis mellifica, Urtica urens, Natrum muriaticum and Dulcamara. Take a 6c dose every 30 minutes, decreasing the frequency as relief occurs. If there is no relief after six doses the medicine should be changed (see also p.116).
- **Herbal remedies** include calendula, chickweed and aloe vera ointments for sore, dry or itchy skin, and camomile lotion to relieve inflammation. But remember that you may be allergic, or sensitive, either to the plants themselves or to the other constituents of a commercial preparation.
- **Chinese medicine** recommends cooling foods, such as sunflower seeds, aubergines (eggplants), lettuce and tofu, but always check with your doctor before taking Chinese herbs.
- **Naturopaths** suggest eating plenty of raw foods and excluding sweet ones, including honey and dried fruit.

WHAT YOU CAN DO

1 If you are certain that you have urticaria, take an antihistamine (from your doctor or pharmacist) and/or use one or more of the home remedies (see box). Consult your doctor if your symptoms persist for more than two weeks or if you develop other symptoms, such as wheezing, joint pains or a fever. If you experience any swelling around the face, lips, tongue or throat, take an antihistamine, if available, and seek immediate medical help. See also **anaphylaxis** (see p.13).

p.13

2 Identify the cause, if possible, and avoid it. Common causes include:
- A recent infection: the urticaria will disappear as this resolves.
- Recently started medication: stop taking it and consult your doctor.
- A food item or drink taken in the 24 hours preceding an attack.
- Being stung or bitten by an insect or animal such as a jellyfish.
- Recent contact with plant sap.
- Exposure to the sun or a sunlamp, or extreme heat or cold.
- Emotional upset.

3 Strengthen your immune system by improving your diet (see pp.106–13) and **reducing stress** (see p.122).

Part 3

4 Consider adopting a **low salicylate diet** (see p.72), or avoiding foods that contain or release **histamine** (see p.73) or contain other **additives** (see p.38).

pp.38, 72–3

CAUSES

Urticaria occurs when specialized cells, known as mast cells, release powerful chemicals, including histamine, following exposure to an allergen. The allergen responsible in any particular case can be difficult to establish.

Although the rash is often brief, some people are unlucky enough to have a form of chronic urticaria that comes and goes over months or even years. This can be triggered by **food allergy** or **intolerance** (see p.10), by specific chemicals in food, such as **salicylates** (see p.72) or **histamine** (see p.73), or occasionally by recurrent **thrush infections** (see p.44).

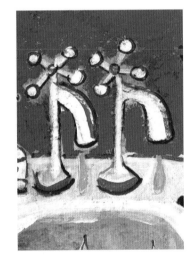

Allergies in the mouth

There are two types of allergy that can affect the mouth. The first is known as oral allergy syndrome, which is similar to urticaria, and the second is contact allergic stomatitis, a condition very like contact allergic dermatitis.

ORAL ALLERGY SYNDROME (OAS)

The symptoms, which are usually mild at first, include itching or tingling of the lips, mouth and throat, followed by the formation of blisters and swelling of the mouth and throat.

CAUSES

Symptoms usually start within 30 minutes of eating raw vegetables or fruit. At first only one or two foods are involved, but the sensitivity may spread to other foods, either in the same botanical family (see pp.76–9) or unrelated (see p.130). The syndrome is uncommon and, although almost everyone who develops OAS has a pollen allergy, very few people with a pollen allergy develop OAS.

In food allergy different foods are involved, including fish, peanuts (groundnuts) and certain medicines, such as aspirin. Food allergy also affects parts of the body other than the lips, mouth and throat.

SIMILAR CONDITIONS

'Pineapple mouth'
a condition whereby an irritant chemical contained in pineapple causes burning and redness of the lips and surrounding skin.

'Citrus mouth'
in which similar symptoms are caused by contact with limonene, an oil contained in the skin of citrus fruit, dill, caraway and celery.

WHAT YOU CAN DO

If you find yourself developing symptoms of OAS, avoid swallowing any more of the food you are eating, and seek urgent medical attention. Your doctor will be able to confirm the diagnosis by arranging skin and blood tests. With the exception of carrots, a recurrence of symptoms can usually be avoided by cooking the food responsible. This changes the nature of the molecule to which the body is reacting. **Individual medical advice**, however, is essential.. (see pp.136–7)

pp.136–7

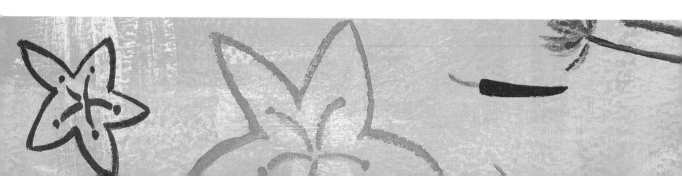

CONTACT ALLERGIC STOMATITIS

With this condition, there is often very little obvious change for your doctor or dentist to see, but symptoms can be unpleasant and include pain, numbness, a burning sensation and loss of taste. Unlike contact allergic dermatitis, which can spread to other parts of the body (see p.24), the effects of allergic contact stomatitis remain confined to the mouth, strictly where direct physical contact has occurred. Fortunately the condition is rare, as in most people saliva dilutes and washes the allergens away.

CAUSES

Allergens that can cause contact allergic stomatitis include:

- toothpaste, including any dyes they contain
- mouthwash
- medication applied within the mouth, such as lozenges for sore throats and ulcers
- fillings, crowns, dentures etc.
- lipstick
- nail varnish, if you bite your nails
- nickel, from sucking jewellery
- foods

WHAT YOU CAN DO

1 See your doctor and/or dentist for a correct diagnosis. The condition is rare and a number of other more common problems need to be excluded.

2 Try to identify the cause of your contact allergic stomatitis and then avoid it. In some cases, **neutralization** or **EPD** (see p.137) may be helpful.

p.137

MOUTH ULCERS

Viral infection is the most common cause of mouth ulcers, but they can also be a problem if you suffer from certain mineral and vitamin deficiencies, Crohn's disease, ulcerative colitis or coeliac disease. If you do not have these conditions, but suffer recurrent bouts of mouth ulcers, you may find you get relief by altering your diet, because in some people mouth ulcers appear to be caused by food intolerance, especially in those who are prone to other allergic conditions. Gluten appears to be the most likely culprit, so it's worthwhile excluding wheat, rye, barley, corn (maize) and oats first. If your ulcers do not improve, try following the **Diet Plan** in Part 2.

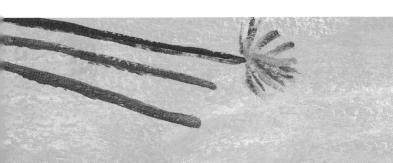

Contact allergic dermatitis

Contact allergic dermatitis is an allergic response to a substance that has been in close contact with the skin. Molecules of the allergen are absorbed into the body and sensitize all parts of the immune system. As a result, the dermatitis may spread if the original substance is touched again, or you may find that the dermatitis develops on distant areas of skin.

CAUSES

Contact allergic dermatitis can occur at any age, from infancy onwards, but it is most common in young adults. The condition can flare up quite suddenly, as a reaction to virtually any substance. You may even find that you develop a reaction to a substance that has been in contact with your skin for years without previously causing any problem. As a result of this, it can be extremely difficult to determine what is causing contact allergic dermatitis. There are common culprits and these include nickel, perfume, hair colouring, aftershave and cosmetics.

Making an accurate diagnosis of the condition can also be problematical as the appearance of the skin may not differ much from irritant dermatitis. This is a local irritation to the skin that is caused by contact with substances such as soap, detergent, polish, bleach or even, occasionally, raw food.

HOME REMEDIES

Treating skin allergies can be difficult and prevention is often better than trying to cure them. If you have a sensitive skin, or have had eczema in the past, try to minimize the risk of developing further allergic reactions by following a good skin care regime:

- **Avoid exposure to the sun**, and choose sun lotions carefully, as many contain fragrances or other substances that can provoke a reaction. Always test a small patch of skin before you apply the lotion over a large area (see box opposite).
- **Do not allow your skin to become dry.** Exposure to water removes its protective oils, so make showers or baths brief, and take them only when needed. Dry your skin without rubbing it, and be generous in your use of hypoallergenic moisturizers and emollients, especially when the air is dry, either from heat or cold, or after spending time in an air-conditioned room.
- **Use mild, acidic soap** to protect the slight natural acidity of your skin, or rinse using a dilute solution of vinegar (60ml/ 2 fl oz per 1.2 litres/2 pints water).
- **Eat a healthy diet** (see pp.106–13) and reduce the stress in your life (see p.122).
- **Always keep your doctor informed** if your skin has shown an allergic reaction, especially to a drug or, if you need surgery, to latex (rubber) or a metal.

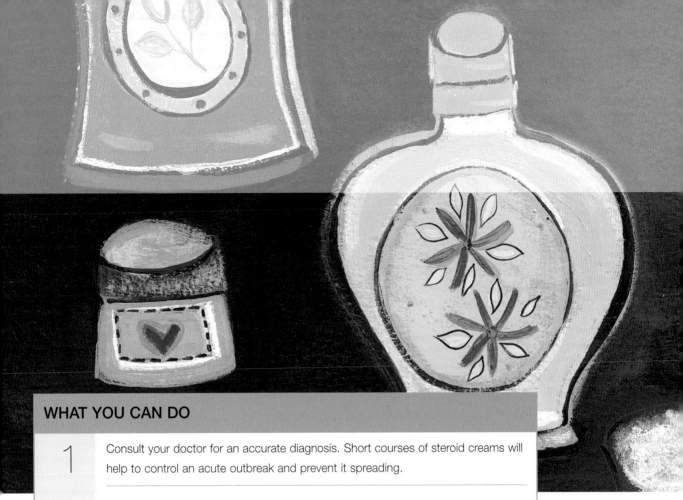

WHAT YOU CAN DO

1 Consult your doctor for an accurate diagnosis. Short courses of steroid creams will help to control an acute outbreak and prevent it spreading.

2 In the longer term, avoidance of the allergen is the mainstay of treatment because the allergy does not usually go away, and for this the allergen must be recognized, usually by patch testing on the skin. As there are so many candidates, you may need to do your own patch testing by taping suspect substances, such as a piece of material or a leaf, to your skin with hypo-allergenic tape. However, this should never be done with a strong chemical or when your skin is red, sore or broken. Do not apply a patch test to a small child without first discussing this approach with your doctor. If the site begins to itch remove the tape, as the test is positive. Otherwise wait 48 hours and inspect the skin; the test is positive if the area is raised or red. If the test is negative, replace the tape and check again after a further 48 hours. For liquids, such as perfumes, or aromatherapy oils, place a little behind your ear and leave the area unwashed for 48 hours. If the skin becomes red or itchy, the test is positive. If you have a sensitive skin, use one of these methods before changing to a new product, such as hairspray, cosmetics, hair dye, aromatherapy oil, etc.

3 Desensitization with **homeopathy** or **neutralization** are possible other options, if the cause is known (see p.117, p.137).

A reaction to cosmetics is a common cause of contact allergic dermatitis, even cosmetics you may have been using trouble-free for many years.

pp.117, 137

Allergies affecting the eyes

These allergies usually affect the skin of the eyelids and around the eye, and the conjunctiva – the membrane that lines the inner surfaces of the eyelid and covers the white part of the eye. Both are likely to have been in contact with the allergen.

ALLERGIES AFFECTING THE EYES

In allergic conjunctivitis, the eyes appear bloodshot, tears flow, the upper and lower eyelids are painful and swollen, and the eyes itch or burn. Normally, both eyes are affected simultaneously and, nearly always, **allergic rhinitis** (see p.28) occurs at the same time.

CAUSES

There are numerous triggers that can set off a bout of allergic symptoms affecting the eyes. These triggers include the following:

- Airborne allergens, such as **pollen** (see opposite); **house-dust mites** and their faeces (see p.19); **mould** spores (see opposite); **animal dander** and **feathers** (see p.14); **household sprays** and **chemicals** (see p.126).
- Contact allergens, such as cosmetics; contact lenses and their cleaning and storage solutions; paper tissues; adhesives used to attach false eyelashes; nickel in eyelash curlers.
- Ingested allergens in food, although these always cause other symptoms elsewhere in the body at the same time.

WHAT YOU CAN DO

1   Seek medical advice, unless you are certain of the diagnosis. In severe cases, your doctor may prescribe steroid drops, but using these requires close medical supervision. Antihistamine drops are safer, but you may start to react to the constituents of any eye drops. You can also take antihistamines by mouth, and/or **homeopathic medicines** (see p.116).

p.116

2   Identify your allergens and avoid them whenever possible. They may be obvious, for example, symptoms may start after you change your eye make-up; or seasonal, being caused by, for instance, grass pollen. If they aren't obvious, you may need to use **skin patch tests** (see p.25) or ask your doctor to arrange **skin prick tests** (see p.136). **Homeopathic desensitization** (see p.117) or **neutralization** (see p.137) are potential options when avoidance is impossible.

pp.25, 117, 136–7

Dealing with pollens and mould

FOR QUICK RELIEF

Splash your face with cold water or cover it with a damp cotton cloth.

You can often reduce, or even eliminate, the symptoms of allergic conjunctivitis and rhinitis by taking simple measures to avoid the allergens that cause them, such as pollens and mould spores.

Pollens are in the air from late winter to late autumn. If your symptoms are seasonal, find out which pollens are in your area at the time you have problems (see p.27 and p.28). In addition:

- **Keep all windows shut**, and use air filters at home, work and in your car.
- **When you go out wear wrap-around sunglasses** to protect your eyes, also a scarf over your hair, nose and mouth. Avoid problem plants and, during the grass pollen season, take note of the pollen counts and forecasts provided by the media.
- **Consider creating a lo-allergy garden** (see p.128).
- **After being out, remove pollen** by rinsing your hair, changing your clothes, and washing any furry pets that have been outside.

Mould spores are at their most concentrated in the atmosphere from late summer to autumn, decreasing markedly after the first frosts. Moulds can flourish throughout the year, however, in warm, damp conditions, such as those found in modern, hermetically sealed, centrally heated houses. You can reduce your contact with them by:

- **Airing the house every day**, using extractor fans in kitchens and bathrooms, and covering pans that contain boiling water. Also use a dehumidifier if necessary.
- **Drying your clothes out of doors.** If you use a tumble dryer, vent it to the outside.
- **Cleaning the seals round refrigerator doors** regularly, and throwing out old food.
- **Placing a layer of sand on top of the soil** of pot plants and watering from the bottom.
- **Removing mould from shower curtains,** tiles and around window frames by using a solution of either bicarbonate of soda (baking soda) or borax (1 dessertspoon in a bowl of warm water).
- **Prevent dampness penetrating your house,** for example, from leaking gutters.
- **Avoiding areas outside with high mould counts** – near deciduous trees in wet weather, near freshly raked leaves and newly turned compost heaps, the countryside at harvest time and during spring ploughing, and anywhere just before a thunderstorm.

Pets also carry mould, see p.14.

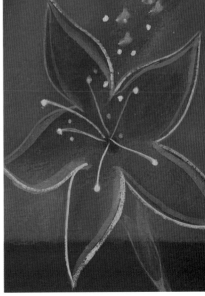

Allergies affecting the nose

Allergic rhinitis is the medical term used to describe an inflammation of the lining of the nose caused by an allergy rather than an infection, such as the common cold.

The symptoms of allergic rhinitis include a 'runny' nose and sneezing, which often occurs in bouts of several sneezes. The nose, palate (roof of the mouth), and sometimes the ears, may be itchy. When the nose is not discharging, it may feel blocked because the tissues are swollen. Often, **allergic conjunctivitis** occurs at the same time (see p.26).

You may need to distinguish allergic rhinitis from the non-allergic kind, which can occur when you eat spices or hot food, drink caffeine, or are exposed to irritant chemicals, such as tobacco smoke or perfume. A runny nose is a side effect of a number of medicines, so if your symptoms begin after you have just started a new prescription you should consult your doctor.

HOME REMEDIES

If you know that pollens are the cause of your rhinitis, smearing some petroleum jelly inside your nose can be very effective. This is because pollen grains split and release their aggravating contents after landing on a watery surface, not a greasy one. Always make sure you reapply the cream after blowing your nose.

What you eat during the pollen season may increase your sensitivity as the allergens in pollen are similar to those found in some foods. Most people find that they can eat the problem foods without any difficulties at other times of the year. If your symptoms improve after avoiding the foods listed below, it is worth challenging yourself with each food separately (for advice on this see pp.98–101), as you may find you don't need to avoid them all.

If you react to tree pollens – symptoms occur from midwinter onwards – avoid:
• hazelnuts, celery, carrots, swede (rutabaga), parsnips and potatoes (including peeling potatoes).

If you react to grass and cereal pollens – symptoms occur in early summer – avoid:
• milk (cow's, ewe's and goat's), and all milk products, including cheese and yogurt.
• related cereals: wheat, barley, rye, oats, corn (maize), wild rice.
• other foods: all beans and lentils, including peanuts (groundnuts), soya and soya products, liquorice, tapioca, and senna (which may be present in medication). For **cross-reactions** see p.130.

WHAT YOU CAN DO

1 Treatment, which can be either conventional or homeopathic, should begin as soon as symptoms appear and includes:
- Antihistamines by mouth.
- Steroid nasal sprays: these are both safe and usually very effective when they are used every day, though it may take up to two weeks for symptoms to subside.
- Intramuscular steroid injections: these are usually reserved for severe symptoms that do not respond to the above measures.
- **Homeopathic medicines** (see p.117).

Caution: Avoid nasal decongestants as they can cause rebound swelling and discharge form the nose, making it almost impossible to stop using them, although applying steroid nasal sprays for a couple of weeks usually helps. You then need to decrease the decongestant, one nostril at a time, before stopping it completely. Expect to have a few days of discomfort during this time.

p.117

2 Try to identify your allergens and avoid them (see also **pollens and mould**, p.27), or consider **homeopathic desensitization** (p.117) or **neutralization** (p.137).

pp.27, 117, 137

3 Consider specific dietary options. If pollens cause your symptoms, see home remedies opposite; otherwise consider trying a **low salicylate diet** (see p.72), which may be particularly helpful if you have had nasal polyps, and/or excluding other **additives** (see p.38).

pp.38, 72

4 Alternative therapies that may be alleviate symptoms include **homeopathy** (see p.146) and **aromatherapy** (see p.150).

pp.146, 150

CAUSES

- Airborne allergens, such as **pollen** of all types (see p.27), **house-dust mites** and their faeces (see p.19), **mould spores** (see p.27), **animal dander** and **feathers** (see p.14) and **household sprays** (see p.126).
- Occupational allergens, such as grains and their flours, wood dust, plastics and epoxy resins, latex (rubber).
- Ingested allergens in food and **food additives** (see p.38). Bear in mind that ingested allergens will always cause other symptoms elsewhere at the same time.

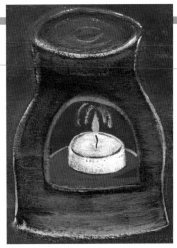

Burning aromatherapy oils can ease symptoms of allergic rhinitis.

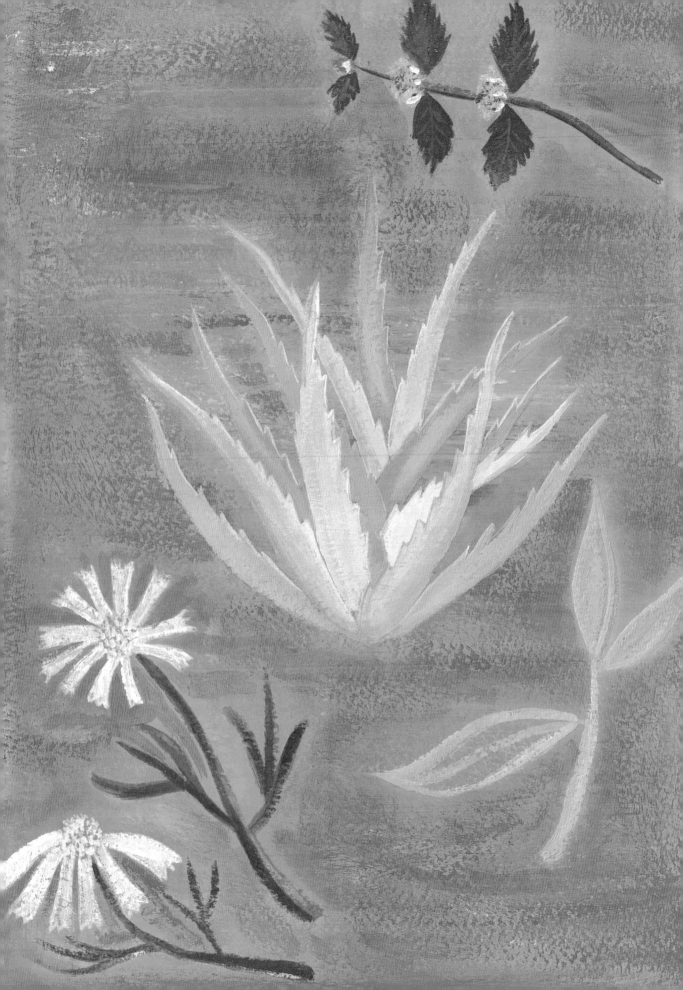

Asthma

Asthma is a Greek word meaning 'to breathe hard', which is the main symptom of the condition. It occurs when the walls of the respiratory passages, the airways, over-react to changes in their environment.

When a person suffers from asthma inhaled allergens or changes in air temperature cause the membranes that line the airways to become swollen and to produce mucus. This causes the tiny muscles in the walls of the airways to go into spasm. Each of these changes causes the airways to narrow and therefore restricts the flow of air. The person affected will suffer shortness of breath, wheezing, coughing and chest tightness.

CAUSES

The underlying causes are uncertain, but we know asthma tends to run in families, particularly those prone to other allergic conditions. Children of low birth weight and those who are over-exposed to **allergens in their first year of life** are most at risk, especially if their parents smoke (see p.131).

If you have a tendency to asthma, it can be set off by exposure to allergic and/or non-allergic triggers. Allergic triggers include:

- Inhaled allergens, such as **house-dust mite** faeces (see p.19), **pollens and mould spores** (see p.27), **animal danders**

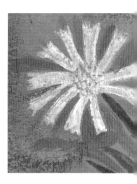

HOME REMEDIES

The Buteyko method, developed by Konstantin Buteyko in the 1950s, is best taught by a practitioner, but if you do not have access to one try the following:

- Sit comfortably in an upright chair. Breathe in, then out and hold your nose. Pause for as long as you can. Try to practise four times a day and adopt a routine of four long pauses, followed by three minutes of shallow breathing and then two medium pauses.
- Breathe through your nose at all times, if possible, and try to avoid gulping air.
- Do not lie down, except to sleep, and, when sitting, try to remain upright.

Herbal remedies can also be beneficial for asthma but avoid steam inhalations, as these can precipitate an attack of asthma. You could try the following:

Roman camomile: add 2–3 drops of the essential oil to a saucer of warm water and leave in your bedroom at night. (Avoid during pregnancy.)

Eucalyptus: place a few drops of essential oil on your pillow, or add 1ml to 25ml of carrier oil for a chest rub.

Aloe vera, taken by mouth, may be beneficial for asthma. In one study, a teaspoonful (5ml) of a 20 per cent solution taken twice a day over 6 months relieved asthma in people who did not require steroid medication.

White horehound: take as an infusion, tincture or syrup.

and **feathers** (see p.14).

- Food and drink, **food additives** (see p.38) and certain medicines, including **aspirin and related medicines** (see p.72), and beta blockers (used to treat high blood pressure).
- Smoky places: 7 out of 10 children in one survey said smoke made their asthma worse.
- **Occupational allergens** (see p.48 and p.126).

NON-ALLERGIC TRIGGERS INCLUDE

- Exercise.
- Changes in temperature, especially going from a warm house into cold air.
- Emotional stress.
- Hormones: many women are more prone to asthma just prior to their periods.

WHAT YOU CAN DO

1 Take your medication as prescribed. Asthma is a serious condition; conventional therapy controls most people's symptoms very effectively and enables children to grow normally. Always talk to your doctor first before changing your medication or embarking on alternative treatment.

2 Try to identify and, if possible, avoid the triggers that cause your symptoms. Conventional skin and blood tests can usually identify allergic triggers, and **neutralization** (see p.137) or **homeopathic desensitization** (see p.117) may help.

pp.117, 137

3 If necessary, **improve your diet** (see pp.106–13), and try to eat foods that contain **magnesium** (see p.113), as this helps the muscles that line the airway to relax.

pp.106–13

4 Do **breathing exercises** (see p.120 and p.124) and/or the **Buteyko method** (see p.31), and take regular, gentle **exercise** (see p.118).

pp.30, 118, 120, 124

5 Consider following a **low salicylate diet** (see p.72) – especially if aspirin makes your symptoms worse – and reducing your intake of **food additives** (see p.38).

pp.38, 72

6 Even if conventional tests are negative, you may obtain relief if you identify and exclude foods to which you are intolerant (see the **Diet Plan** in Part 2). Be aware, however, that asthmatics sometimes experience severe reactions when reintroducing foods, so you will need personal medical supervision.

Part 2

7 Helpful **alternative therapies** include Western herbalism, osteopathy, chiropractic, yoga, acupuncture, homeopathy, hypnotherapy, aromatherapy, autogenic training and biofeedback (see p.140).

Part 4

Genitourinary symptoms

People who have multiple allergies, food intolerance or both, often develop symptoms involving the bladder and genitalia.

Urinary symptoms, such as frequent urination, bladder pain and recurrent cystitis for which no bacterial cause can be found, are sometimes the result of food intolerance. Painful and heavy or irregular periods, pre-menstrual symptoms and, in the older woman, flushing, sweats and other menopausal symptoms can all be symptoms of food intolerance. The genitalia may also become swollen, itchy and/or painful, or a woman may develop a vaginal discharge after coming into contact with an allergen. Common allergens include soap, bath gels and other bath additives, antiseptics and toiletries, traces of biological washing powder left behind after washing, dyes in clothes, the rubber in condoms or diaphragms and the constituents of spermicides. Very occasionally, a woman may also react to her partner's sperm.

WHAT YOU CAN DO

1 **For symptoms involving the bladder**
- See your doctor for conventional treatment if you have problems.
- If tests are negative, consider following the **Diet Plan** in Part 2.

Part 2

1 **For gynaecological problems**
- Adopt a really **healthy diet** for a few months (pp.106–13).
- If your symptoms do not improve, it may be that you have a food intolerance and need to consider the **Diet Plan** in Part 2.

Parts 2 & 3

1 **For genitalia and allergy**
Consult your doctor or dermatologist for a diagnosis and to establish the cause.

2 If no cause is isolated symptoms may improve by eating a **healthy diet** (see pp.106–13).

3 If you are no better after a few months, you may wish to consider the **Diet Plan** in Part 2.

FLUID RETENTION

Excessive thirst is a common symptom in food intolerance. Thirst can cause frequent urination or fluid retention, which worsens when you eat the suspect foods. Some doctors believe that food intolerance causes a change in the body's chemistry, leading to fluid retention. Women can be thirsty, and retain fluid before a period, and it is a common symptom in **hyperactive children** (see p.38) and their fathers, and in people deficient in **essential fatty acids** (see p.110).

Irritable bowel syndrome (IBS)

Some 70 per cent of people who have been told by their doctors that they have IBS can improve or eliminate their symptoms by making dietary changes.

WHAT YOU CAN DO

1 Consult your doctor for a diagnosis. She or he may prescribe conventional drugs to take when the symptoms are particularly severe. Try to avoid antibiotics whenever possible, as **Candida** (see p.44) can occur at the same time.

p.44

2 Dietary changes that are usually recommended include avoiding **caffeine** (see p.73) and increasing the **fibre in your diet** (see p.109) by eating more fruit and vegetables and switching to whole grain cereals. If increasing the whole wheat in your diet or taking a wheat bran supplement makes your symptoms worse, you may be intolerant of wheat so, to test this, it is worth **excluding wheat** from your diet completely for 5–6 days and then challenging yourself with it (see p.98).

pp.73, 98, 109

3 If you think your symptoms may, even partly, be caused by **stress**, take measures to try to reduce it (see p.122). Vigorous **exercise** (see p.118) or simply going for a walk can be useful, as it not only keeps the bowel active but also reduces stress.

Part 3

4 IBS can be caused by a diet that contains too much refined sugar. If you have a sweet tooth it is worth trying to **exclude refined sugar** from your diet for a few weeks. (For a list of foods that contain sugar, see p.57.)

p.57

5 If your symptoms persist even after taking the above measures, following the **Diet Plan** in Part 2 will help you to discover if you have a food intolerance. More than one food may be causing your symptoms, but not usually more than three or four. The most common culprits are wheat or corn (maize), cow's milk and milk products, tea, coffee, onions, potatoes and citrus fruit, but virtually any food can be responsible.

Part 2

6 Helpful **alternative therapies** include naturopathy, Chinese or Western herbalism, massage, yoga, acupuncture, psychotherapy, hypnotherapy, homeopathy, aromatherapy, chiropractic, osteopathy, autogenic training and biofeedback.

Part 4

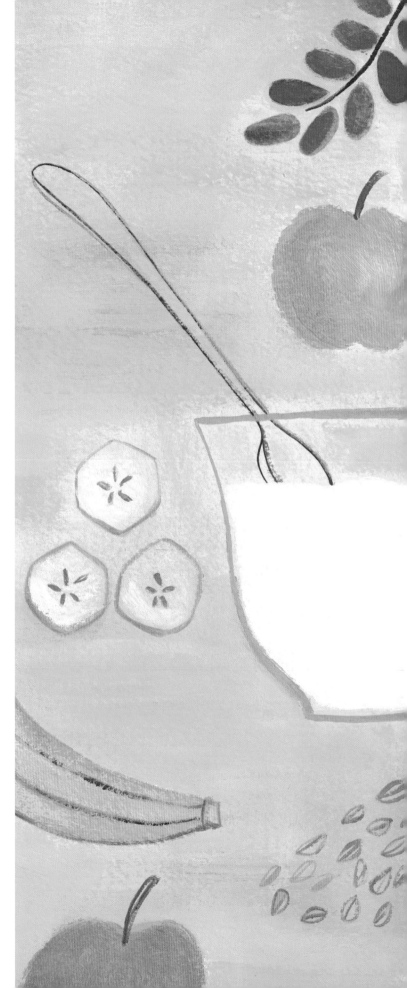

Eating live yogurt and increasing your intake of fibre by eating more fruit can ease symptoms of IBS.

Many people suffer from IBS, but the condition tends to occur most frequently in women during their childbearing years. Symptoms include various combinations of the following:

- **Pain in the abdomen** that appears to be related to the function of your bowel; for example, it may disappear after your bowels have moved, or you have passed wind.
- **Changes to the normal pattern** of opening your bowels, such as increased or decreased frequency, the need to hurry or to strain, the feeling that your bowel is not completely empty.
- **Changes in the composition** of your stools, such as being too hard, or too soft, or variable from day to day.
- **Increased passage of mucus**, either with the stool or on its own.
- **A feeling of distension** or bloating of the abdomen, which may or may not be improved when you pass wind.
- In women, the symptoms are often worse just prior to their period.
- **Various degrees of feeling stressed**, including anxiety and depression.
- **Recurrent thrush infections** (see p.44).

HOME REMEDIES

- Some people benefit from eating **live yogurt** (see p.112) others use **herbal supplements**, especially mint (see p.115).

Any of these symptoms or other changes in bowel action should be discussed with your doctor so that an accurate diagnosis can be made. Other bowel problems can appear to be very similar to IBS, but require different treatment. Blood is not usually present in the stools in IBS but, if you notice any, always consult your doctor as this requires full conventional investigation.

CAUSES

Some doctors believe that IBS is largely a psychological problem, and this can certainly be the case when the symptoms start after an emotional upset, such as bereavement, or during a time of great stress. However, food intolerance is a more common cause, and symptoms usually respond well when the **culprit foods** are detected and temporarily avoided (see Part 2).

GALLSTONE SYMPTOMS

Some doctors have found that identifying and eliminating certain foods can reduce or even cure symptoms apparently caused by gallstones – such as abdominal pain and wind. Adopting this approach can also be effective if these symptoms persist after gallstone surgery. In addition, following the **Diet Plan** in Part 2 may not only relieve symptoms, but can also help with weight loss in cases where it is recommended before surgery can be undertaken.

INFANT COLIC

Milk intolerance is a common cause of the colic that babies can develop at the age of 3–4 months. Symptoms are often relieved by switching to a milk-free formula or, if the baby is being breastfed, by the mother excluding milk from her diet. In both instances professional advice should be sought to ensure that the baby receives sufficient **calcium** (see also p.131).

HOME REMEDIES

- **Rubbing the baby's tummy** or allowing it to lie prone on a firm surface, such as across your knee, may relieve the symptoms.
- **Herbal remedies**, such as drinks containing fennel or camomile, and homeopathic medicines, such as 6–10 granules of Chamomilla 6c or Dioscorea 6c, placed in a teaspoon with a drop of water and administered every 30 minutes, as needed, for up to six doses, may also relieve symptoms.

Weight problems

Intolerance to food and perhaps chemicals can be a reason for being overweight or underweight, since it appears to have a direct effect on appetite, food cravings, fluid retention and also on the way the body controls weight and blood sugar levels.

Food craving is a common symptom in people with a food intolerance. In many cases the foods that are craved are the ones causing the intolerance. Once these are eliminated from the diet, the craving usually disappears. Sometimes chromium and magnesium deficiencies also need to be reversed, either by improving the diet or by taking supplements. Sugar craving, however, can also be a symptom of **Candida** (see p.44) or the result of eating too much **refined sugar** (see p.56 and p.108).

Food intolerance can also cause loss of appetite and weight loss, which usually resolves when the culprits are withdrawn. A long-standing lack of appetite may cause mineral deficiencies, especially of magnesium and zinc, which will need to be corrected, if necessary by taking supplements.

WHAT YOU CAN DO

1 Try keeping a **food, mood and symptom diary** for a few weeks (see p.54). This may help to identify foods that you crave and perhaps have an intolerance to.

p.54

2 Adopt a **healthy diet** (see pp.106–13), in which calories are restricted to about 1500 per day for women and 1800 for men. (These should be increased if weight loss exceeds 1 kg (2.2 lb) per week after the first couple of weeks when fluid is lost.)

pp.106–13

3 At the same time, start an **exercise** programme (see p.118). Aim for 30–45 minutes moderate exercise five days a week. This doesn't have to be taken all at once – a brisk 10–15 minute walk to the shops can be counted. Try also walking up stairs instead of taking a lift; if this makes you too breathless, start by walking down first!

p.118

4 If you follow these measures for 2–3 months without losing weight, you may be intolerant of one or more foods. Following the **Diet Plan** in Part 2 may be helpful.

Part 2

5 In addition to the above, it may be worth reducing your exposure to **chemicals** (see p.48 and pp.126–30), as these can cause food cravings and fluid retention.

pp.48, 126–30

Hyperactivity

Even a mild degree of hyperactivity in a child can cause a lot of disruption, both at home and in school. When a child has severe hyperactivity it is medically recognized as attention deficit hyperactivity disorder (ADHD).

As the name suggests, there are two aspects to ADHD: difficulty in concentration and hyperactivity. These are present to differing degrees. Boys are more likely to be overactive, and so are noticed. In girls, poor concentration may dominate, so despite the presence of learning difficulties the diagnosis may be less obvious. The condition often resolves towards late adolescence, but it may persist into adult life.

CAUSE

The exact cause of hyperactivity is unclear, and many factors have been implicated in the condition, including difficult births and nutrient deficiencies during pregnancy and early infancy. In some cases there is probably also an inherited predisposition, so someone who was affected in childhood may find they encounter the problem again as a parent.

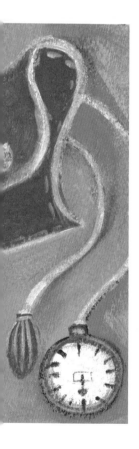

Food intolerance may also be a cause, as many children improve with dietary changes. Even when the hyperactivity is sufficiently severe for a diagnosis of ADHD to be made, research suggests that about a quarter or more of children with ADHD behave normally when they eat a diet that excludes food to which they are intolerant. In addition, a number of others improve enough to allow them to respond better to psychological treatment.

FOOD ADDITIVES

Around 3000 additives are present in modern foodstuffs and medicines. They preserve food, ensuring safety and extended shelf life, and enhance flavour and appearance. To avoid them, you need to check all food labels and enquire about the constituents of medicines.

Virtually any additive can cause symptoms in a susceptible person. The commonest culprits are:

Natural additives: which include substances most likely to cause food intolerance, such as thickeners from wheat or corn (maize) and natural sweeteners/syrup from corn (maize), beet and cane. Both are found in liquid medicines and even tablets. Albumen usually comes from eggs.

Flavourings (E620–3*): the most notorious is monosodium glutamate (MSG), which can cause Chinese restaurant syndrome (flushing, chest tightness and pain, headache and fainting).

Antioxidant preservatives (E320–1*): these prevent fats from going rancid, but can also trigger asthma and urticaria.

Sulphite preservatives (E220–8*): these occur naturally when yeast ferments, but may be added to beer, wine and fruit juice, or used

WHAT YOU CAN DO

1 Begin by keeping a **food, mood and symptom diary** (see p.54) to help you identify possible trigger foods and chemicals.

p.54

2 Avoid food additives (see list of additives opposite), as these are the most common triggers for hyperactive behaviour. Use plain white toothpaste and avoid gel toothpaste as this contains preservatives.

3 Eat a **healthy diet** (pp.106–13) to avoid swings in the level of sugar in your blood.

pp.106–13

4 The next stage for adults is the **Diet Plan** in Part 2. For a child, discuss this approach with your doctor first, as you may need the help of a dietitian to ensure that the diet is adequate for growth.

Part 2

5 Discuss other treatments that might benefit hyperactivity with your doctor. These include behavioural therapy and medication.

6 **Homeopathy** (see p.146) can sometimes be beneficial, but you will need to consult a qualified practitioner, preferably one who is also a doctor.

p.146

in the preparation of seafood, gelatine, dehydrated vegetables, pickles, preserved meats, sausages, fruit salads, dried fruits and green salads, which are sprayed with sulphite preservatives to preserve freshness in salad bars and restaurants. Can trigger asthma, rhinitis and urticaria.

Nitrite and nitrate preservatives (E249–51*): these stabilize the colour of cooked meats, including ham and bacon, and cheese. Can trigger urticaria and headaches.

Benzoate preservatives (E210–8*): these are used in fruit squashes, fruit syrup, fizzy drinks, some vegetables and shellfish. Can occur naturally in honey, and cranberries. Often implicated in ADHD. Can cause urticaria, and possibly eczema and asthma. May affect people who are sensitive to aspirin (see p.72) and/or tartrazine (E102).

Food colourings: Azo dyes (E100–80*): these are found in many foods and medicines. Can be broken down in the gut to form amines (see p.73). Can cause asthma, urticaria, behaviour disturbances, hyperactivity and migraine.

*An 'E' number is given to some, but not all, the additives that are approved by the European Union (EU), and are quoted here as they appear on food labels in the EU.

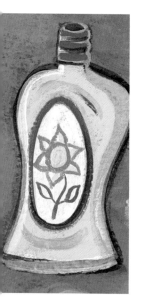

Migraines and food intolerance

Up to one in ten people experience migraine headaches at some time in their lives. The fortunate ones have only one or two episodes in a lifetime, but others may suffer migraine headaches several times a week.

Migraine headaches usually affect only one side of the head and are experienced by the sufferer as a throbbing or pounding sensation. Their onset is sometimes signalled by alterations in the senses, such as smelling or hearing things that other people do not, tingling sensations or numbness in the arms or face, especially in the upper lip. A common warning is an alteration in vision, known as an aura, in which the person sees areas that sparkle with bright colours or assume a zigzag appearance. These symptoms are thought to be caused by a narrowing of the blood vessels supplying the brain.

After half an hour or so the blood vessels dilate again and become stretched, causing pain. The throbbing or pounding sensation is the result of the pulsation of blood caused by the heart beating and altering the pressure inside the blood vessels. It is usually so intense that the person needs to lie quite still in a dark quiet place. Nausea and vomiting are often present; some people report that they pass large amounts of urine as the migraine clears. For many people, sleep cures the symptoms.

WHAT CAUSES MIGRAINE?

Migraine is sufficiently common and disabling to have resulted in extensive research. It is probably best regarded as a symptom that can be produced by a number of different changes in the biochemical activity of the body. As the tendency to migraine runs in families, these changes are probably to some extent inherited. There are, however, several immediate triggers to migraine headaches, which have to be identified for any one individual, and avoided whenever possible. These triggers include:

- **Food intolerance** (see p.11).
- **Eating foods that contain or release histamine** (see p.73).
- **Food additives** (see p.38), such as MSG or nitrates.
- **Withdrawal from caffeine** (see p.73) or certain painkillers used to treat migraine, such as ergotamine or those that contain caffeine.
- **Stress**, exhaustion or emotional changes, including excitement.
- **Too much or too little sleep.**
- **Hormonal changes in women**, including taking the birth control pill.
- **Muscle tension** (e.g. grinding the teeth), eyestrain or poor posture.
- **Weather**, for instance changes in barometric pressure or exposure to the sun.
- **Minor head injury.**

WHAT YOU CAN DO

1   There are many types of headache with many different causes so it is important to consult your doctor for a correct diagnosis. If you grind your teeth, consulting your dentist may also be helpful.

2   Consult your doctor about any medication you are taking. If you are having frequent migraines, it could be that the trigger is simply the withdrawal of the medication each time an attack wears off.

3   Try to identify your migraine trigger(s), see opposite. You may find a **food, mood and symptom diary** (see p.54) is helpful, as it has been suggested that 80–90 per cent of people who suffer migraines also have some form of food allergy or intolerance. The diary may also help you decide whether you would benefit from reducing the foods that contain or release **histamine** (see p.73), or whether **food additives** are a problem (see p.38).

pp.38, 54, 73

4   Look at your lifestyle. Can you **reduce your stress** (see p.122) or increase the amount of **exercise** you take (see p.118)?

pp.118, 122

5   Eat a **good diet** (see pp.106–13). The tendency to migraines may be increased if your diet is deficient in B vitamins, magnesium, and essential fatty acids, or contains excessive animal fat.

pp.106–13

6   Consider following the **Diet Plan** in Part 2, unless you have lost the use of an arm or leg or have experienced severe visual disturbances during the course of a migraine in the past. In such cases experienced medical supervision is needed, since severe migraines can occur when foods are reintroduced.

Part 2

7   Helpful **therapies** in Part 4 include homeopathy, Western herbalism, massage, chiropractic, osteopathy, acupuncture, shiatsu, hypnotherapy, biofeedback.

Part 4

Feeling tired all the time

There are numerous reasons why you may feel tired all the time; it may even be the result of medication you are taking. In any event, it is essential you see your doctor for an individual diagnosis, since diseases that have tiredness as a major symptom, such as diabetes, anaemia or heart disease, all require conventional treatment.

Other common causes of tiredness, such as depression and stress, are less easily diagnosed, either by laboratory tests or on physical examination. Poorly controlled levels of sugar in the blood can also cause tiredness, and may be a factor in causing depression.

Chronic tiredness was first recognized as a key feature in food intolerance as long ago as 1930 and since then many doctors have confirmed this observation. Tiredness can also be present if you have recurrent episodes of **thrush** (see p.44), or have **chemical sensitivity** (see p.48).

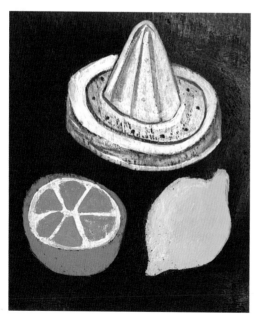

Increase your intake of vitamin-rich fruit and vegetables to combat tiredness.

HOME REMEDIES

Easy dietary changes to introduce when you are feeling tired include:

- **Eating and drinking plenty of fruit and vegetables and vegetable juice**, as they contain magnesium, potassium and phytochemicals (see p.109). (Avoid too much carrot or beetroot juice as these contain high levels of sugar.)
- **Eating as many different foods** as possible, this helps to reduce symptoms caused by food intolerance.
- **Excluding alcohol**, caffeine, nicotine, refined sugar and white flour, they make the tiredness worse and your body has to use up vital nutrients to deal with them.

CHRONIC FATIGUE SYNDROME

The existence of chronic fatigue syndrome (CFS) was not formally recognized until the late twentieth century. The basis on which doctors can make the diagnosis remains controversial, and there is no specific test to confirm diagnosis.

CFS usually occurs after a viral infection, especially glandular fever, but often it has no obvious cause. Only about a quarter of people who have long-term

WHAT YOU CAN DO

1 See your doctor for a diagnosis.

2 Improve your **diet** (see box opposite) so that you supply your body and immune system with the nutrients they need for healing. Even if you feel totally exhausted, it really is worth the effort of trying to make a few small improvements. Once you are comfortable with these you will hopefully feel well enough to do a little more (see pp.106–13). In addition, make sure you eat at regular intervals, and in a relaxed environment whenever possible.

pp.106–13

3 Try to reduce **stress** (see p.122), and make time to include a gentle, gradually increasing, **exercise** programme (see p.118), such as **tai chi** (see p.121).

p.118, 121, 122

4 Make sure you have enough rest and try to establish a regular sleep pattern. **Learn how to relax** (see p.124). Sleep is often disturbed in CFS and may improve with a low dose of a conventional antidepressant drug (even if you do not feel particularly depressed). If the prescribed dose makes you too sleepy, ask your doctor to reduce it. Some people are extremely sensitive to medication but can avoid the sleepiness, yet achieve better sleep, with the dosage that might be given to a small child.

p.124

5 Consider taking mineral and **vitamin supplements**, especially vitamin C, B vitamins, zinc and magnesium (see Part 2). If possible, it is best to obtain professional individual advice about appropriate dosages.

Part 2

6 If you remain tired 4–6 weeks after introducing the above measures it is possible you have food intolerance and should consider the **Diet Plan** (see p.52).

p.52

7 Consider trying an **alternative therapy.** Helpful therapies include massage, yoga, psychotherapy and acupuncture (see Part 4).

Part 4

debilitating tiredness suffer from CFS, but around half of those who do also have a history of allergic disorders, such as hay fever, asthma and eczema.

Related conditions include fibromyalgia (muscle pain) and **chemical sensitivity** (see p.48). In both these conditions many of the symptoms are similar to those reported in CFS, and they may be particular forms of CFS. Sometimes the sufferer is found to have low levels of magnesium and in such cases intra-muscular supplements may be helpful.

The Candida problem

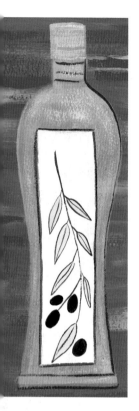

Candida albicans is a type of yeast, more commonly known as thrush. A normal inhabitant of the intestine, it can cause active infection when it occurs in places other than this, such as on the skin, or in the vagina or mouth. More widespread and serious infection can affect people who are seriously debilitated, from illness, including cancer, or as a result of extreme old age.

There is little scientific support for the idea that an overgrowth of Candida within the intestine itself can cause symptoms. However, it is recognized that the microbes that normally control the amount of Candida can become unbalanced after taking antibiotics. There is also evidence to suggest that if this imbalance persists, then the sufferers intestine may become 'leaky', resulting in incompletely digested foods being absorbed, leading to stress of the immune system.

Some doctors believe that the resulting symptoms are best called 'dysbiosis', because it is likely that Candida is not always the cause, even though the symptoms may often include recurrent episodes of thrush infection. Alternative practitioners, however, and the

HOME REMEDIES

Seek extra help from proven Candida fighters:
- Helpful foods include normal culinary use of: raw garlic, live yogurt (see **probiotics**, p.112), ginger, oregano, basil, rosemary, thyme, peppermint and cold-pressed extra-virgin olive oil.
- Useful supplements include caprylic acid, grapefruit seed extract, oregano oil, *Pseudowintera colorata* and Pau d'arco (as a supplement or made into a tea).
- Helpful herbal preparations include plants that contain a substance called berberine: goldenseal (*Hydrastis canadensis*), barberry (*Berberis vulgaris*), Oregon grape (*Berberis aquifolium*) and goldenthread (*Coptis chinensis*).
- Eat food that is rich in **fibre** (see p.109) and consider supplementing your diet with **fructo-oligosaccharides** (FOS, see p.112).

Ideally, Candida fighters should be taken under professional supervision but, if this isn't possible, follow the manufacturer's instructions, taking a break every month to see if you need to continue taking them. If either you, or your partner, suffers from frequent attacks of thrush, wash underwear at 80°C (176°F) to eliminate thrush from the fabric and reduce the risk of reinfection.

WHAT YOU CAN DO

1 If you think you may have a Candida problem, try to have the diagnosis confirmed by a doctor. Even if your doctor is reluctant to confirm the diagnosis, they will be able to exclude other possible conditions and, if necessary, to prescribe conventional anti-thrush medication.

2 Improve your **diet** (see pp.106–13). Consider taking a sugar-free, yeast-free multi-mineral and vitamin supplement, some extra vitamin C, and one or more Candida fighters (see home remedies). Keep your bowels regular with psyllium or linseeds (flaxseeds), taken with plenty of water. If your symptoms have not improved after three months, consider following the **Diet Plan** in Part 2.

Part 2, pp.106–13

3 Take plenty of rest. Consider starting a **stress management programme** (p.122) including gentle **exercise** (p.118), that increases as you begin to feel better.

pp.118, 122

general public, frequently use the term 'Candida problem' when faced with these symptoms.

Clearly there is much work to be done to understand this puzzling condition, particularly as it has become more common over the past 20 years. Its features include:

- **Chronic fatigue**, loss of energy, poor concentration.
- **Indigestion**, distension and bloating.
- **Altered bowel function**, such as increased frequency or constipation, passage of mucus, and stools that are either harder or softer than before.
- **Muscle and joint pain.**
- **Itching around the anus** and, in women, recurrent vaginal thrush, or cystitis, in which no microbe can be identified as the culprit.

- **Alterations in the immune system**, causing frequent infections, the development of new allergies, increased symptoms from pre-existing allergies, decreased tolerance of chemicals, such as perfume, cigarette smoke, household cleaning agents, or alcoholic drinks.
- **Previous use of steroid medicines** (e.g. for asthma or arthritis), the birth control pill, or frequent or long-term courses of antibiotics.
- **Craving for sweets**, sugar, carbohydrates or yeast.

ANAL ITCHING

Anal itching can have a number of causes, including thrush infection and food intolerance. If symptoms persist after conventional diagnosis and treatment, try the **Diet Plan** in Part 2.

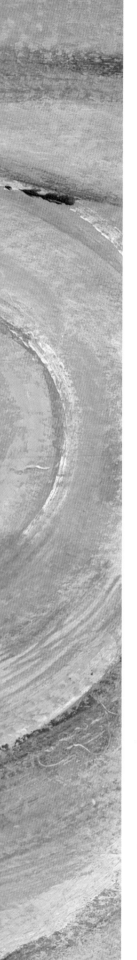

Arthritis can be the result of food intolerance

If you go to a bookshop or library to look for a book on an appropriate diet for painful joints you are likely to find several, all offering conflicting advice. This reflects the fact that the foods that cause intolerance and aggravate arthritis vary from person to person.

Arthritis is a condition causing inflammation of the joints, the symptoms of which are pain and swelling, causing stiffness and limited movement. One of the major problems with a dietary approach to the condition is the fact that the progress of the disease can vary depending on the type of arthritis you have. In many types, symptoms come and go of their own accord, and it is easy to assume that the dietary changes you have adopted are the reason for the improvement. Many doctors believe that dietary changes have no role to play in controlling the symptoms of arthritis, whilst others believe that food intolerance is a common contributory factor.

CAUSES

The underlying causes of arthritis are not generally understood. Conventional treatment may be unavoidable, but it acts to suppress symptoms rather than treating the root causes, which may or may not include food intolerance.

Use your **food, mood and symptom diary** (see p.54) to detect the non-food causes of joint pain, so that you can take steps to avoid them. They include:

- **Inhaled allergens.** These are uncommon in hot, dry climates, so if your symptoms improve when you have a holiday in a warm place, house-dust mites (see p.19) or mould spores (see p.27) may be responsible. If you are always better away from home, in any climate, it may be the pets (see p.14) or chemicals (see p.48) that you have left behind that are causing the problem.
- **Alcoholic drinks.** If your joints are worse after drinking beer, wine or cider, you may be intolerant of yeast or have a Candida problem (see p.44). Spirits are less likely to cause symtoms, unless you are intolerant of a component, such as a grain or potatoes, or added sugar or syrup.
- **Cigarette smoke.** Tobacco comes from the nightshade family (see p.78) and can cause symptoms if you are intolerant of members of that family. If you are a smoker you may find giving up is easier when you exclude foods from this family from your diet.
- **Food additives** (see p.38). These are excluded in the mini-elimination diet stage 1 (see p.58).

WHAT YOU CAN DO

1   Start a **food, mood and symptom diary** (see p.54) and, because joint pain can have so many causes, include a column to note the weather, where you were and what you were doing (see causes, opposite).

p.54

2   Improve your **nutrition** (see pp.106–13), and eat a diet that is low in saturated fat, sugar and salt. Make sure that you obtain sufficient essential fatty acids, copper and zinc. Extra pantothenic acid (vitamin B5) can be helpful in rheumatoid arthritis and vitamin E in ankylosing spondylitis, but it is best to discuss taking these with your doctor first. Do not smoke or drink excessive alcohol.

pp.106–13

3   If you have osteoarthritis of the weight-bearing joints, especially of the hips and knees, your joints are likely to benefit greatly if you lose any extra weight (see p.37).

p.37

4   Take gentle exercise, but with care (see p.118). Exercise often relieves stiffness, and keeps the joints moving fully. However, it is best to avoid running or walking, which may stress your weight-bearing joints, particularly if you have osteoarthritis of the hips, knees or ankles – swimming and cycling are better. Acutely inflamed joints in rheumatoid arthritis should only be moved very gently. If in doubt, seek individual advice from either your doctor or a physiotherapist.

5   Consider food intolerance. Start by excluding the most common culprits: dairy products, grains, coffee, nuts, fruits with pips, and the nightshade family (see p.78). If this does not help, follow the **Diet Plan** in Part 2 of this book. If you have rheumatoid arthritis, you may be able to save time by going directly to the elimination diet outlined on p.94, as improvements can be slow and are difficult to assess on the other diets.

p.52, 78, 94

6   Helpful **alternative therapies** include homeopathy, herbalism, massage, yoga, acupuncture, hydrotherapy and hypnotherapy (see Part 4).

Part 4

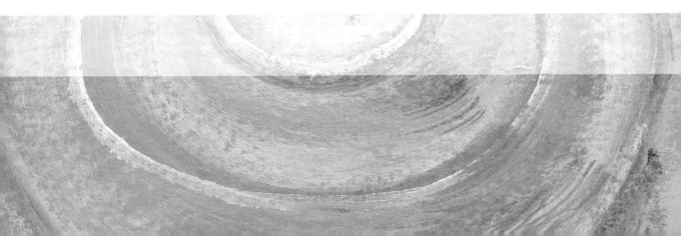

Chemical sensitivity

Millions of new chemicals have been created during the past 50 years, at least 10,000 of which are in regular daily use. Exposure to these chemicals does not cause problems for most people unless the level is high enough to cause poisoning.

Doctors who specialize in environmental medicine believe that, in certain people, long-term exposure to low doses of man-made chemicals causes a form of sensitivity or intolerance. This exposure to chemicals can make the person feel unwell when, later on, they come into contact with the same chemical or chemicals, and often when they are exposed to other chemicals and allergens as well.

A similar reaction can occur when a person is exposed to a single dose of a chemical, when the dose is high enough to cause poisoning. Symptoms will show when the person has not completely recovered from the exposure and they can vary from day to day.
They include fatigue, disturbed sleep, nausea, mood changes, headaches, painful joints and muscles, disturbances of memory, inability to concentrate, palpitations and breathing too fast or too deeply.

Unfortunately, obtaining help if you think you are sensitive to chemicals can be difficult. Many doctors dismiss the idea of chemical sensitivity, not least because the symptoms vary greatly and are difficult to confirm. It is not possible, for example, to prove to someone that you have a headache or 'can't

ALLERGIES AND CHEMICALS
Research suggests that inhaling certain chemicals affects the immune system, increasing the likelihood of it producing an allergic reaction. Other chemicals appear to act as allergens or to have a direct toxic effect. There is increasing recognition that indoor pollution can often be more severe than that found outside.

Problem chemicals include:
- Nitrogen dioxide, from car exhausts and from burning gas for cooking or heating,
- Formaldehyde, from cigarette smoke and a wide range of new furnishing and fittings.
- Volatile organic compounds (VOCs), the term used to describe the cocktail of chemicals released from cleaning agents, paints, photocopying machines, furniture glues and varnishes.

think'. However, because the severity of your symptoms seems to depend on the 'total load' of chemicals entering the body, you may feel better and have more energy if you avoid chemicals as much as possible, and improve your diet. Such changes can strengthen the immune system and help the body deal with the chemicals you cannot avoid.

WHAT YOU CAN DO

1 **Chemical sensitivity**

If you think you have chemical sensitivity, try to confirm the diagnosis by finding a doctor who has an interest in environmental problems. Even if this is not possible, you should discuss your symptoms with your doctor to exclude the possibility that your symptoms have another cause.

2 Eat a **healthy diet** (pp.106–13). If you are not able to obtain personal professional advice about taking **food supplements**, consider starting a sugar-free, yeast-free multi-mineral and vitamin preparation (see p.112).

pp.106–13

3 Try to identify the causes of your symptoms by starting a **food, mood and symptom diary** (see p.54). For example, your symptoms may only occur at home.

p.54

4 Reduce your overall exposure to **chemicals and other allergens** in your home and workplace (see p.19, p.27, pp.126–30). It may be best to start in your bedroom, as you spend a third of your life there. Try the **mini-elimination diet** stage 1 (p.58), as it excludes many **food additives** (p.38).

p.19, 27, 38, 58, 126–30

1 **Allergy in the workplace**

Suspect a workplace allergy if your symptoms started soon after you took up new employment or your conditions of employment changed, or when the pattern of your symptoms changes, being present at work or when following your hobby but not at other times. It is important to identify the cause of your symptoms, as avoidance is often the best way to control them. Your doctor, occupational physician or dermatologist will be able to help you, and to suggest treatment where this is appropriate.

2 Check the section in this book that covers your symptoms (see box).

SYMPTOMS OF A WORKPLACE ALLERGY

By definition a workplace allergy is one that is caused by exposure to a chemical or other allergen at work, but allergies can also be caused by exposure to similar substances when they are used in a hobby.

Every year thousands of people have to change their job or hobby because of allergy. The symptoms can include **rhinitis** (see p.28), **conjunctivitis** (see p.26), **urticaria** (see p.20), **contact allergic dermatitis** (see p.24), **asthma** (see p.30) and, rarely, **anaphylaxis** (see p.13).

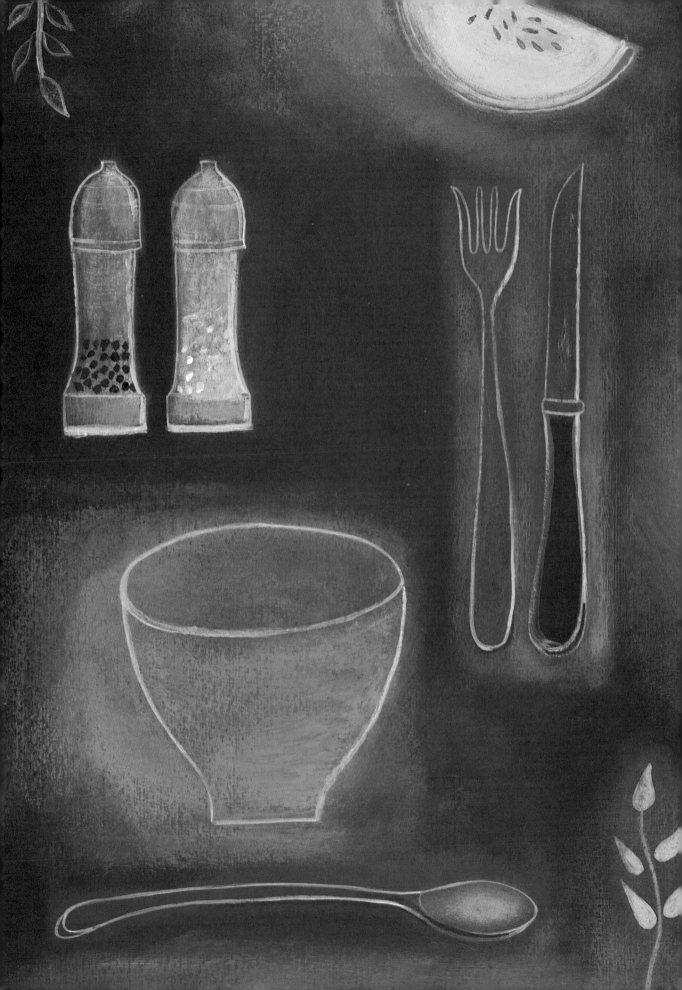

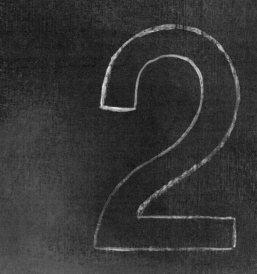

2

The
diet plan

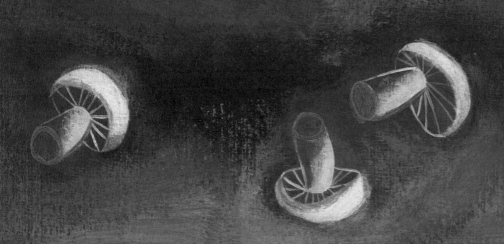

The Diet Plan

The aim of this Diet Plan is to help you identify any foods to which you are intolerant, by following a step-by-step progression. If you have been directed in Part 1 to the Diet Plan, you should begin with the mini-elimination diet, and then proceed to the next stage according to how you are progressing.

PREPARING FOR THE DIET PLAN

The Diet Plan is based on both eating plenty of fresh whole foods and avoiding food additives, preservatives, flavourings and colourings. To succeed, you will need to get into the habit of reading food labels. You may be surprised by the amount of sugar contained in 'ready-made' meals. Starting the Diet Plan can seem daunting, but with a little planning – for example, writing yourself daily menus for the first week – it is possible to avoid having to do too much extra work. As you begin to feel better, you will discover you have more energy and organizing your diet will become easier. If you are 'addicted' to foods that are excluded, you may need to find ways of avoiding temptation, such as banishing them from your kitchen.

ORGANIC OR NON-ORGANIC?

Whether or not you choose organic food is often an economic decision, as organic food is generally more expensive than non-organic. It is true that there are some people who are so sensitive to chemicals that opting for organic produce improves their symptoms considerably. For the majority, however, eating the recommended 2–4 portions of fruit and 3–5 portions of vegetables each day is of greater value than eating organically grown produce in smaller amounts.

CHECK YOUR STORE CUPBOARDS

As you prepare to start the Diet Plan, take a close look at the food in your cupboards. Any items containing additives should either be put away or given away as, initially, your diet needs to be completely additive-free. You may also need to remove items from your freezer – many convenience foods contain additives, and as a result are unsuitable for the Diet Plan. One way of avoiding being a slave to the stove is to make your own 'convenience' foods by cooking enough food for two or three meals, and freezing portions for future use.

SHOPPING GUIDE

Unfortunately, some vitamins are lost during storage, so you will probably need to make more than one shopping trip each week in order to ensure your fruit and vegetables are fresh. Frozen vegetables are a useful standby for emergencies or for when you are tired or in a hurry, but make sure they contain no additives, sugar, for example, is often added to frozen peas. Avoid canned foods, as the lining of some cans is a phenol resin, that contaminates food slightly and people can be sensitive to it.

Meat and fish should be bought in their original unprocessed form, but they can be frozen, if they are of good quality. Try to avoid all processed foods, even those labelled as being free of 'artificial' additives, as food labels are not necessarily accurate, and the food may contain items that are excluded in the Diet Plan. Although cheese, milk and eggs frequently cause food intolerance, they are allowed in the early stages of the Diet Plan, except for very ripe cheeses, which may contain **histamine** (see p.73).

Most dry, staple foods can be eaten in the early stages of the plan, as they do not contain additives, though white grains and flours, including pasta and rice, should be replaced with whole grains and whole grain products, as these are richer in essential minerals and vitamins. Sweet biscuits are excluded, but rice cakes, oat cakes and whole grain crispbreads are permitted at first. Check that your breakfast cereal does not contain any sugar or sweeteners, even honey.

Buy dried, rather than canned, beans and lentils, for the reason given earlier. Lentils cook very quickly, and are filling and nutritious when used in sauces or added to pasta and soups. Although beans have to be soaked first, you can bulk cook them and freeze the extra in appropriately sized packs for future use. If you find they give you wind, **sprout them** for a few days before cooking (see p.92). See also lectins p.73.

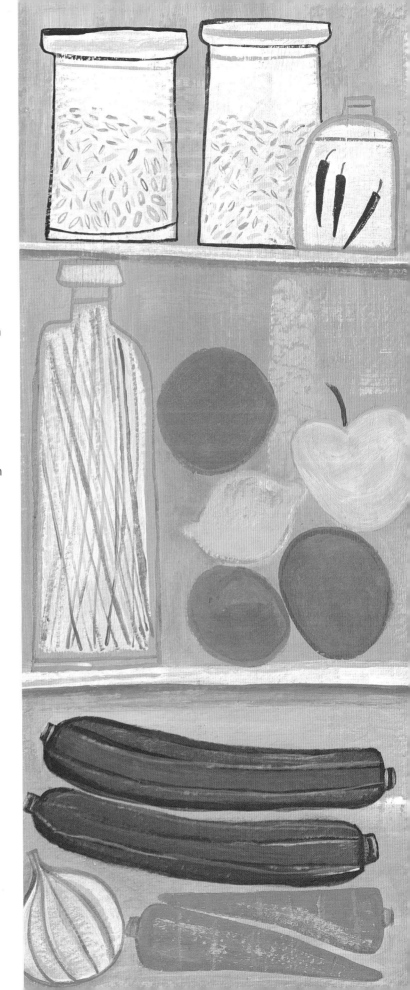

Before you start

Take courage; very few people need to complete all stages of the Diet Plan. The majority find that they feel considerably better and their symptoms have been alleviated after completing the two stages of the mini-elimination diet.

Even these stages require some effort, however, and most people will want to avoid undertaking them more than once. This means spending some time in preparation. The most important first step is to go back to Part 1 of this book, and ensure that you have tried the other measures suggested for your condition. This may sound obvious, but if your condition improves, even slightly, by following these measures you should continue them while on the Diet Plan to obtain the best possible results. You may not have to do so for ever, but suddenly discontinuing them at the start of making dietary changes can mean that any changes in symptoms will be difficult to interpret.

As you may need to follow the Diet Plan for 2–3 months, it is preferable not to start just before Christmas, a holiday or a big family celebration. You will obtain the best results if you try to be as strict as possible, so you should avoid times when this will be difficult. Do not regard the waiting period as time wasted; many people benefit more than they would have thought possible from simply continuing with a **healthy diet** (see pp.106–13), just as others find that they learn more about how food affects them by keeping a diary (see below).

Once you have decided to try the Diet Plan, consult your doctor and describe your

KEEP A FOOD, MOOD AND SYMPTOM DIARY

Keeping good records is an essential part of the Diet Plan. Maintaining a food, mood and symptom diary will help you to detect which foods are causing your symptoms and to gauge your progress. If possible, begin the diary a week or so before starting the Diet Plan. It is often difficult to remember exactly how you felt a few weeks ago, and your diary will jog your memory and help you to appreciate the progress you have made, even if it seems slow. The diary does not need to be elaborate – an exercise book is perfectly adequate – though you will need to draw three columns in order to record:

• Date and time.
• What you eat or drink .
• How you feel at the time you eat or drink, and any symptoms that occur at other times.
  Measure and record your weight each day. This is best done when you get up in the morning, after having emptied your bladder, whilst you are still either naked or in your nightclothes.

symptoms. Ask for any necessary check-ups, both to exclude a different diagnosis and to rule out other conditions that would lead your doctor to advise against your following the Diet Plan. On the whole, it is best to avoid taking unnecessary medicines while following the Diet Plan, so consult your doctor about this if you are taking **prescription medicines**, including, in the case of women, the birth control pill (see p.94).

STOP SMOKING

There is little point in trying to sort out your health while continuing to poison yourself with your own cigarette smoke, or in the case of passive smoking, other people's smoke.

WITHDRAWAL SYMPTOMS

Initially, when you stop eating foods to which you are intolerant, your symptoms may become worse or you may develop new symptoms, such as tiredness, depression, aching muscles or headaches. These symptoms can last up to ten days, but the most severe are usually over by the fourth day. In some people, weight loss occurs as the body loses water. Although these symptoms can be unpleasant, they can be

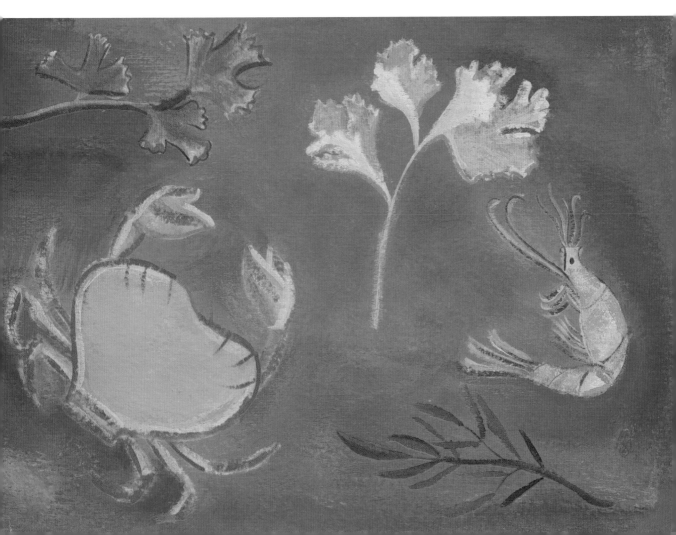

THE DIET PLAN

viewed as a very good sign, as once they have cleared you are likely to feel much better.

You can reduce the severity of these withdrawal symptoms by:

- **Excluding caffeine** (see p.59 and p.73) and sugar (see p.57) before starting the Diet Plan.
- **Drinking extra water** (see p.106).
- **Taking extra rest.**
- **Taking extra vitamin C**, for example 250mg, three times a day (but not at bedtime as it may keep you awake).
- **Having plenty of warm (not hot) baths** or showers if your sweat smells unpleasant.

EXCLUDING REFINED SUGAR

Many people find withdrawal from refined sugar an uncomfortable experience. The body absorbs refined sugar quickly, but because excess amounts can be damaging, it also produces a surge of insulin to control the level of sugar in the blood. To some extent the body becomes used to the amount of sugar we eat each day, with the result that, when sugar is suddenly withdrawn, too much insulin may be produced for a few days until the body adapts to the new regime. In addition, for people who are intolerant of sugar, there is an element of addiction, as we seem to crave the foods to which we are intolerant. For both reasons the desire for sugar is likely to be strong.

You can either opt to get the discomfort over and done with at once by just excluding sugar, or you can prolong the experience, but have

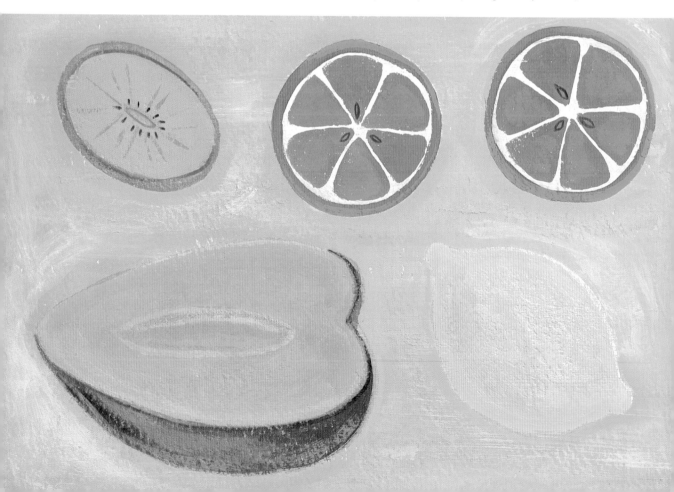

less acute symptoms, by gradually decreasing it. Eating more whole grain foods, beans and lentils can alleviate symptoms, as they help to stabilize the level of sugar in your blood. If you become desperate, eat 85–115g (3–4oz) of fruit (not juice), choosing something that releases its sugar slowly, such as an orange, plum, apple, pear, grapefruit or cherries.

THE DIET PLAN IF YOU ARE A VEGETARIAN

If you are a vegetarian or vegan, it is important that you obtain sufficient protein when following the Diet Plan. The animal proteins eaten by vegetarians are usually derived from milk and, sometimes, eggs. Unfortunately, these are often the very foods that are implicated in food intolerance and, as a result, they are excluded at certain stages of the Diet Plan. Apart from soya beans, quinoa and millet, vegetable sources of protein do not contain all the **amino acids** (see p.107) that

VEGETABLE SOURCES OF PROTEIN

Whole grain cereals: such as wheat, barley, oats, rye, corn (maize), rice, quinoa, millet, buckwheat

Pulses (legumes): such as all types of peas, beans and lentils, peanuts (groundnuts)

Nuts: such as hazels, almonds, pecans, macadamias, brazils, walnuts, hickory nuts, butter nuts, pine nuts

Seeds: pumpkin, sesame, sunflower

vegetarians need, so it is important that they eat protein from a minimum of two sources at least twice a day, if not at every meal.

Vegetarians and vegans should not attempt the full elimination diet without individual professional advice, as decisions as to which protein-containing foods to include need to be taken on a personal basis.

FOODS TO AVOID

Foods that contain sugar:
- **White and brown sugar**, golden (corn) syrup, molasses, maple syrup, malt
- **Barley sweetener** (macrobiotic sweetener)
- **Jam**, including 'no added sugar' jam, marmalade, jelly
- **Chutneys and pickles**
- **Cakes, biscuits, ice cream, puddings**
- **Chocolate, other sweets** and confectionery, including cough and throat lozenges
- **Fizzy drinks, fruit squash, cordials**
- **Any food containing corn syrup, dextrose, glucose, maltose, sucrose, fructose or lactose** (except when it is in milk and milk products)
- **Baked beans**, including those labelled as containing 'no added sugar'
- **Peanut butter**, unless 'sugar-free'
- **Ready-made** soups and meat pies
- **Some medicines**, such as syrups and sugar-coated pills; if necessary, check with your pharmacist

The mini-elimination diet plan
STAGE 1

The mini-elimination diet is a two-stage diet. It is a structured approach to excluding the foods most likely to cause food intolerance.

During stage 1, sugar, caffeine, alcohol and many added chemicals are excluded. Unless you have already excluded **sugar** and **caffeine** (see p.57 and p.73), this will signify a big change to your diet, and your digestion may need time to adapt. If you experience **withdrawal symptoms**, see the advice given on pp.55–6.

If you already eat few processed foods and have a low intake of caffeine, refined sugar and alcohol, you may wish to progress immediately to stage 2. You will obtain the best results if you are as strict as possible as far as the diet is concerned; if you deviate from it, you may find that your symptoms return.

FOODS YOU CAN EAT

- **Any fresh, unprocessed meat, fish or eggs.**
- **Beans and lentils:** if you find they give you wind, sprout them before cooking (see p.73 and p.92).
- **All fresh fruit and vegetables**, except pineapple and papaya.
- **All grains**, including rice, rye, oats, barley, corn (maize), buckwheat, wheat, millet and quinoa; for unusual grains see p.68.
- **Whole grain breads**, crispbreads and biscuits, such as rice cakes and oat cakes.
- **Home-made, sugar-free pastry**, flatbreads, crispbreads (see p.63) and drop scones (see p.62). Use wholemeal flours.
- **All seeds and nuts.**
- **Milk, butter, hard cheeses** and other milk products.
- **Vegetable juices** and unsweetened, fresh, diluted fruit juices.
- **Herbal teas**, either commercially produced or made by infusing herbs or spices.

FOODS TO AVOID

- **Caffeine:** no tea, coffee, chocolate or cola drinks (including decaffeinated preparations) or painkillers that contain caffeine. If you normally have caffeine several times a day, reduce your intake gradually over a week or two, to avoid withdrawal symptoms. Herbal teas are permitted, but not maté, redbush, jasmine, gunpowder or other green teas.
- **Sugar:** see the list on p.57.
- **Alcoholic drinks:** including alcohol-free beers and wines, and any food cooked in alcohol. Vinegar and sugar-free pickles can be eaten once or twice a week.
- **All artificial sweeteners:** read food labels carefully, as sweeteners are often added to processed foods, such as fruit yogurts and sugar-free drinks.
- **All foods containing additives:** colourings, preservatives, flavour enhancers, flavourings, thickeners, emulsifiers and stabilizers. Some E-numbers are natural ingredients of food, but at this stage it is simplest to exclude them all (see also p.38), which means avoiding bacon, ham, corned beef and all 'smoked foods'.
- **Very ripe or blue cheeses.**
- **All take-away and fast foods.**
- **Foods that make the intestine leaky** (see p.44), including highly spiced foods, raw pineapple, papaya, aspirin, ibuprofen and other non-steroidal anti-inflammatory painkillers. But consult your doctor before stopping prescribed medicines.
- **Bran:** if you normally take extra bran to avoid constipation, decrease the amount gradually as you increase your intake of fruit and vegetables. If necessary, take linseeds (flaxseeds) or psyllium, with plenty of water.

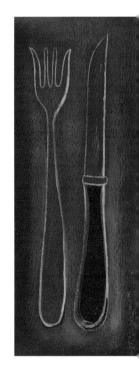

WHAT TO DO NEXT

After a month, you can assess your progress. How are your symptoms?

Much better: Gradually reintroduce the foods that you have excluded (pp.98–101).

A little better or about the same: If you think you have a **Candida problem** (see p.44) go to the next stage of the **Candida diet** (p.70) otherwise progress to **stage 2 of the mini-elimination diet** (see p.60).

Worse: If you have cut down from large intakes of caffeine, alcohol or sugar, continue with stage 1 for another couple of weeks to make sure that you are not still experiencing withdrawal symptoms. If you have added new food items to your diet, you may be reacting to these. Exclude them one at a time, strictly for five days, then eat a reasonable portion to see whether you develop symptoms or your **pulse rate increases** (p.98). Continue to exclude any to which you have reacted. Then maintain stage 1 for another 2–4 weeks, after which you can reassess your progress. If your symptoms have not improved at all, return to your normal diet and consult your doctor.

pp.98–101

pp.44, 60, 70

p.98

The mini-elimination diet plan
STAGE 2

Stage 2 of the diet is more restrictive, but there are still plenty of foods you can eat. Aim for as varied a diet as possible, but be very strict about adhering to it and maintaining your diary. If you continue to lose weight after the first day or so, when retained water may be lost, you are probably not eating enough. Instead of bread, try drop scones or crispbread (see p.62 and p.63), but use oil rather than butter for the chestnut and buckwheat crispbreads. If you dislike ewe's and goat's milk, try nut or rice milk. Also, feel free to add flavourings, such as salt or fresh fruit juice.

FOODS YOU CAN EAT

- **Any fresh, unprocessed meat or poultry**, except beef and chicken (see p.76).
- **Any fresh fish** (though not from the mollusc or crustacean families, see p.78)
- **Beans, lentils and their flours** (except those made from soya).
- **All vegetables**, except members of the nightshade and lily families (see p.78). If you are hungry or losing weight, you may have to be adventurous and try new vegetables, especially starchy ones such as parsnips, pumpkins and sweet potatoes.
- **All fruits**, except the citrus family (see p.76), papaya and pineapple.
- **Buckwheat, quinoa, sago, tapioca, arrowroot, chestnut, rice** (but not wild rice), including any flours or pastas made from them. (See also p.68 for substitutes for excluded foods.)
- **Any nuts and seeds** that you do not normally eat frequently.
- **Goat's and ewe's milk**, cheese and yogurt, coconut milk and milks made from nuts you eat infrequently (see recipes opposite).
- **Filtered water** or good quality non-carbonated spring water, preferably from glass bottles.
- **Vegetable juices** and unsweetened, fresh, diluted fruit juices from allowed fruit.
- **Olive or rapeseed (canola) oil** for cooking; olive, sunflower, safflower oil for dressings.
- **Sea salt, spices and herbs** in moderation.

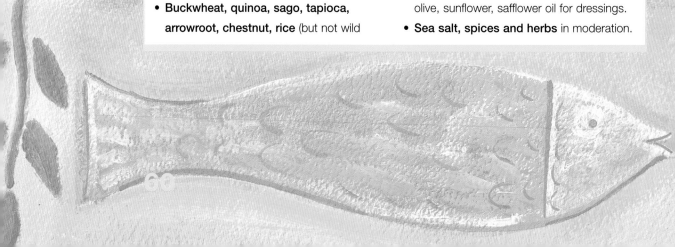

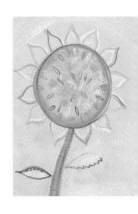

MILKS

Nut milks

These are very easy to make, but vary in texture and taste according to the type of nut used. Soft nuts, such as pine nuts, walnuts, pecans, almonds and pistachios, make relatively smooth, easily puréed milks. Harder nuts, such as hazels and brazils, require longer liquidizing, which may take its toll on your processor. As a rough guide, allow 200ml (7fl oz) water for every 115g (4oz) nuts, and skin them where possible. To make cream reduce the amount of water by a third.

Oat milk

Oat milk tastes rather like liquid porridge – brilliant if you like porridge but, if you don't, you may prefer to pour it on your cereal rather than drink it neat.

25g (1oz) rolled oats
575ml (1 pint) water
pinch of salt (optional)
1tsp honey (optional)

Put the oats in a pan with the water and salt and bring to the boil. Simmer for 10 minutes, then purée in a liquidizer or food processor. Sweeten with honey, if necessary, and chill.

Rice milk

The length of time it takes to make rice milk varies according to the type of rice used. The recipe below uses whole grain brown rice, so reduce both the amount of liquid, and the cooking time, if you use white rice.

25g (1oz) whole grain brown rice
850ml (1½ pints) water
pinch of salt (optional)

Put the rice in a saucepan with the water and salt and bring to the boil. Simmer, uncovered, for 40–60 minutes or until the rice is quite soft. Purée in a liquidizer or food processor, then chill.

FOODS TO AVOID

Continue to exclude the same foods as you did in stage 1, plus the following:

- All members of the grass family (see p.78), including their flours and pastas, and any foods containing 'added starch'
- Cow's milk and milk products
- Soya and soya products
- Eggs
- Foods containing yeast, fermented foods and mushrooms (see p.70)
- Peanuts (groundnuts), and peanut oil (groundnut oil)
- Any food you eat either daily or most days, and foods that you crave
- Any food that you suspect may be the cause of your symptoms, or to which a close relative is intolerant
- Tap water

Many foods you need to exclude are present in manufactured foods, see p.67 for those that often contain hidden wheat, corn (maize), soya, milk, eggs and peanuts (groundnuts).

Breakfast suggestions

Breakfast can often be a difficult meal during stage 2 of the mini-elimination diet, but ideas include:

- quinoa porridge with permitted milk and fruit
- carrot juice and buckwheat noodles with stewed tomatoes and grated goat's/ewe's cheese
- drop scones or crispbread with stewed fruit
- leftover rice, fried with onions and spices, plus fruit salad

DROP SCONES

55g (2oz) gram (chickpea) flour
55g (2oz) brown rice flour
1 level tsp wheat- and gluten-free baking powder
pinch of bicarbonate of soda (baking soda)
pinch of cream of tartar
1tbsp of allowed oil
75ml (3fl oz) allowed milk/water

MAKES ABOUT 15

Sift the flours into a bowl and stir in the other dry ingredients. Make a well in the centre, pour in the oil and milk or water and, using a wooden spoon, beat until you have a smooth batter. Set aside for at least 15 minutes. Wipe a piece of oiled kitchen paper over a griddle or non-stick frying pan, then heat the pan until it begins to smoke. Using a small ladle, drop spoonfuls of the mixture on to the pan – three or four at a time. Cook the scones for about a minute, or until small bubbles appear, then flip them over and cook on the other side. Serve at once, either alone or with grilled bacon, maple syrup or whatever else you fancy – and is allowed.

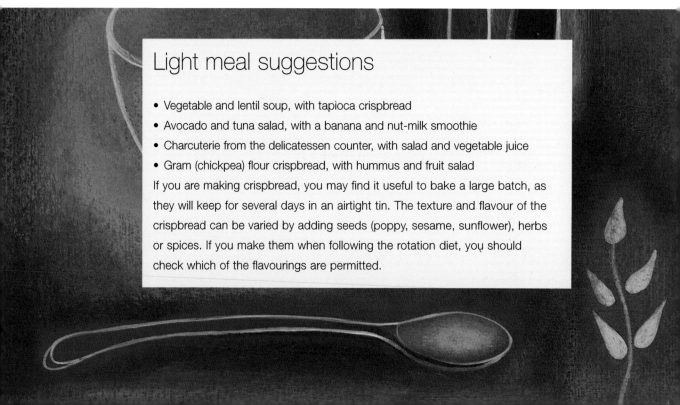

Light meal suggestions

- Vegetable and lentil soup, with tapioca crispbread
- Avocado and tuna salad, with a banana and nut-milk smoothie
- Charcuterie from the delicatessen counter, with salad and vegetable juice
- Gram (chickpea) flour crispbread, with hummus and fruit salad

If you are making crispbread, you may find it useful to bake a large batch, as they will keep for several days in an airtight tin. The texture and flavour of the crispbread can be varied by adding seeds (poppy, sesame, sunflower), herbs or spices. If you make them when following the rotation diet, you should check which of the flavourings are permitted.

CRISPBREADS

Since the flours used here are made from different carbohydrates (starches), they react in different ways when they are cooked. You need to vary the amount of liquid and the cooking times according to the flour used.

The recipes here are suitable for stage 2 of the mini elimination diet, but can also be used in the rotation diets (see pp.74–90).

MAKES ABOUT 5

Preheat the oven to 200ºC (400º F), gas mark 6.

Rub or stir the fat into the flour, then add the water and the salt, if using. Knead gently into a ball. Lightly flour a work surface and roll out the mixture quite thinly. Using a glass, press out 4–6 crispbreads and transfer them to a floured baking tray.

BUCKWHEAT CRISPBREAD (Rotation diet days 1 & 2)

55g (2oz) buckwheat flour
2tbsp olive oil
1tbsp water
pinch of salt (optional)

Bake for 15 minutes.

CHESTNUT CRISPBREAD (Rotation diet days 1 & 2)

55g (2oz) chestnut flour
2tbsp sunflower oil
2tbsp water
pinch of salt (optional)

Bake for 10–12 minutes.

TAPIOCA CRISPBREAD (Rotation diet days 3 & 4)

55g (2oz) tapioca flour
1tbsp rapeseed (canola) oil
1tbsp water
pinch of salt (optional)

Bake for 11–12 minutes.

GRAM (CHICKPEA) FLOUR CRISPBREAD (Rotation diet days 5 & 6)

55g (2oz) gram/chickpea) flour
1tbsp sesame oil
1tbsp water
pinch of salt (optional)

Bake for 10 minutes.

CORNFLOUR CRISPBREAD (Rotation diet days 7 & 8)

55g (2oz) cornflour
1tbsp corn (maize)/hazelnut oil
1tbsp water
pinch of salt (optional)

Bake for 10–12 minutes.

Main meal suggestions

- Stir-fried pork with assorted vegetables, bean sprouts (see p.92) and rice or quinoa
- Venison with red cabbage and roast parsnips
- Grilled fish with baked sweet potato and green beans
- Buckwheat pasta with roast lamb and broccoli

LAMB WITH SWEET POTATO AND SPINACH

2tbsp olive oil
1kg (2 ¼lb) sweet potato,
   peeled and thinly sliced
255g (9oz) fresh spinach,
   washed throughly
3 large sprigs fresh rosemary
sea salt and freshly ground
   black pepper
half leg of lamb, weighing
   approximately 1kg (2 ¼ lb)

SERVES 4

Preheat the oven to 180°C (350°F), gas mark 4.

Pour the olive oil into the bottom of a heavy-based casserole, just large enough to accommodate the lamb, and cover with the sweet potato. Roughly chop the spinach and spread over the sweet potato. Lay two of the sprigs of rosemary over the spinach and season lightly. Sit the lamb on top of the vegetables, lay the final sprig of rosemary on top, then add enough water to reach three-quarters of the way up the lamb. Cover and bake for 1 hour 20 minutes.

Serve either from the casserole or remove the lamb to a dish and spoon the vegetables and cooking juices around it. Serve alone or with another allowed vegetable.

SALMON WITH CHICORY, LEMON GRASS AND COCONUT MILK

2tsp arame
300ml (½ pint) coconut
   milk
2 heads endive (chicory)
4 pieces of lemon grass
4 salmon steaks
salt and freshly ground black
   pepper

SERVES 4

Soak the arame in the coconut milk for 10 minutes. Meanwhile, finely slice the chicory and then lay it in the bottom of a pan just large enough to hold the four salmon steaks. Lay the lemon grass over the chicory, then place the steaks on top. Lightly season the coconut milk and pour it, together with the arame, over the salmon. Cover the pan and cook gently for 15–20 minutes or until the salmon is cooked. Carefully remove the steaks from the pan, lay them on a warmed serving dish, spoon the chicory and cooking juices over the top and serve at once with jasmine rice and a green salad.

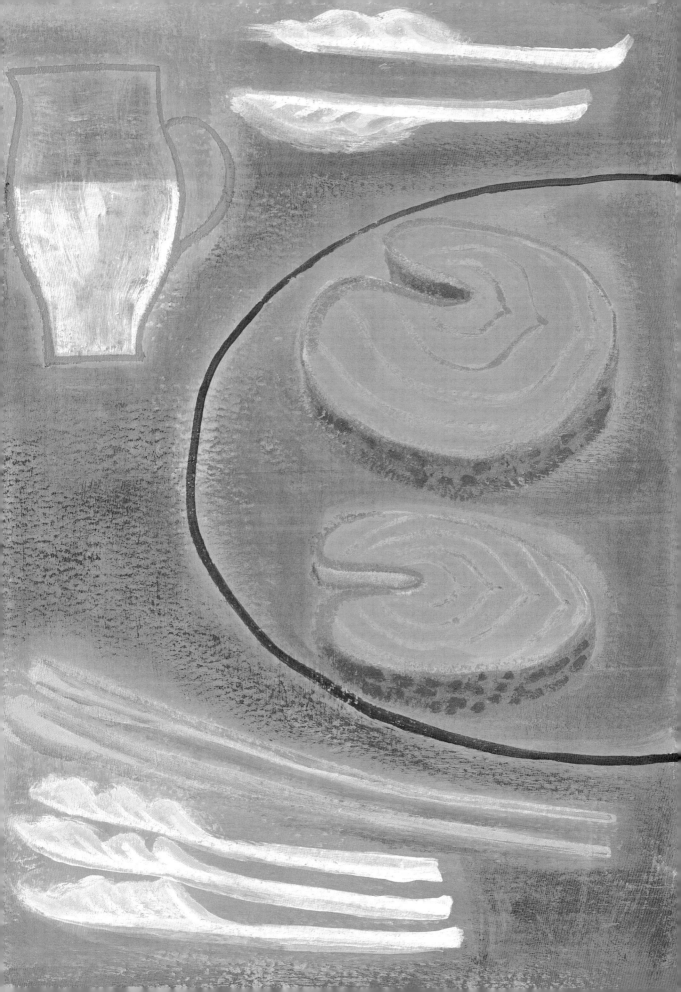

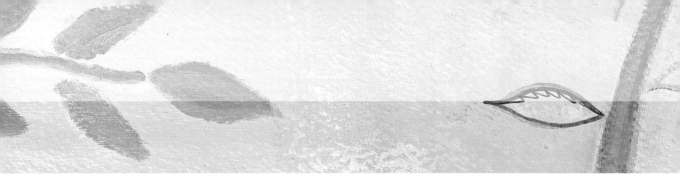

BAKED VEGETABLES

2tbsp olive oil
4 small beetroot, scrubbed
4 small Jerusalem artichokes, trimmed
   and scrubbed
2 pieces of okra, topped and tailed
   and sliced thinly
2 handfuls of green beans, trimmed
   and sliced
2 medium courgettes (zucchini), thickly sliced
25g (1oz) dried sea vegetable (dulse, arame
   or kombu)
1tsp dried dill
4 artichoke hearts, frozen
2tbsp pumpkin seeds
sea salt and freshly ground black pepper
a handful of fresh parsley, roughly chopped

SERVES 4

Preheat the oven to 190°C (375°F), gas mark 5. Pour the oil into an ovenproof dish just large enough to hold all the vegetables and add the beetroot, Jerusalem artichokes, okra, beans and courgettes (zucchini). Mix together well. Sprinkle over the sea vegetable and dill and about 4tbsp water. Cover tightly with foil and bake, stirring periodically, for about 40 minutes or until the vegetables are nearly cooked. Remove from the oven and add the artichoke hearts and pumpkin seeds, then bake for a further 15 minutes. Season to taste and serve sprinkled with parsley.

WHAT TO DO NEXT

Now a month has passed you can assess your progress. How are your symptoms?

Much better: gradually reintroduce the foods that you have excluded (see p.98). p.98

Better but some symptoms remain: you have probably excluded most of the foods causing you problems but there may still be some others giving rise to symptoms. Test the major foods (see pp.98–101) so that you can broaden your diet fairly quickly. Then look through your food diary for items you have been eating throughout and exclude them one at a time for five days at a time before you challenge yourself with them. If you seem to be intolerant of many foods, consider progressing to the rotation diet. pp.98-101

About the same: if this is the case, you either do not have any food intolerance or you are intolerant to so many foods that exclusion is not a viable option. Go to the rotation diet (see p.82) p.82

If you were better but are now getting worse again: this is rare, but suggests that you could be becoming intolerant of new foods. To reduce this problem, switch to the rotation diet (see p.82). p.82

Hidden foods

Many of the foods that are frequently responsible for food allergy or intolerance are contained in manufactured foods. However, if the amount used is small an additional problem is that they may not be included on the label. This list of hidden foods cannot be comprehensive, but will provide some guidance.

EGG is found in cakes, biscuits, puddings and their pre-prepared mixes; in the glaze applied to breads; in egg pasta and noodles; pancakes; meringues; ice cream; sweets; instant coffees; in chocolate and other flavourings used in milk drinks; mayonnaise, salad cream and sauces; wines and beers; baking powder; icing; lecithin. On labels, egg often appears as vitellin, livetin, ovovitellin, ovomucin, ovomucoid and albumin.

SOYA is used to make bread and vegetable oil, some types of textured or hydrolysed vegetable protein, lecithin and many vegetarian ready-meals. Also soya milk, margarine, ice cream, miso, tofu and soy sauces.

PEANUTS (GROUNDNUTS) The oil may be present in vegetable oils, cosmetics, nipple creams and vitamin D preparations. The nuts are often used as a substitute for other nuts.

CORN (MAIZE) is used to make corn oil and other vegetable oils, which are used in the manufacture of crisps and margarines. Cornflour (cornstarch) is used as a thickener and may be present in foods containing starch or baking powder. Sugar is also extracted from corn (maize) and is found in foods that contain glucose, dextrose and golden (corn) syrup, including soft and alcoholic drinks. The gum on stamps and envelopes, and 'vegetable gum' in food may also be made from corn (maize).

YEAST AND SUGAR For foods containing yeast see p.70; for those containing sugar see p.57. Other food preservatives, flavourings, colourings and additives are listed on p.38.

MILK is present in any food containing whey, casein, lactose, lactate, lactalbumin, milk solids or milk fats. Some tablets and inhaled medicines contain lactose. Note that ghee is clarified butter.

WHEAT is found in most baked foods, such as bread, cakes, biscuits, pastas and croutons; also in wheat-based cereals; cereals and crispbreads that contain wheat bran or wheatgerm; processed meats such as sausage; foods with a crumb or batter coating; stuffing; stock cubes, gravy, baking powder; many canned foods and pepper powder. Oatcakes may contain wheat, as may some brands of porridge oats. Ingredients labelled cereal binder, filler or protein may contain wheat, as may foods containing starch, unless the label specifies 'cornflour'; 'gluten' is also often derived from wheat.

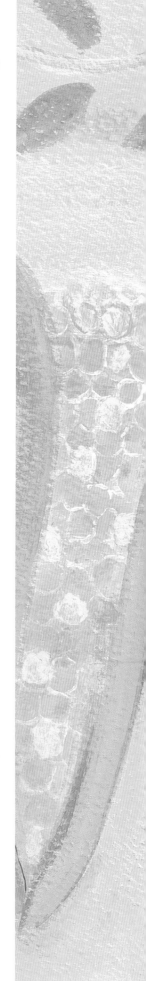

Choosing and using substitutes for excluded foods

Staples such as wheat, eggs and cow's milk can often cause food intolerance. It is important to introduce replacements when staples are excluded from the diet.

GRAINS TO REPLACE WHEAT

The following grains provide energy as well as being good sources of protein and minerals.

Amaranth does not contain gluten. The flour is useful for cakes and biscuits, and the grain can be cooked as a cereal, or added to stews or soups. The grain tastes better if it is toasted in a dry pan for a few minutes before being boiled.

Quinoa needs to be rinsed before being cooked, to get rid of its bitter taste. You can cook it as a porridge or use it as a substitute for rice.

Athough buckwheat contains some gluten, most people who are sensitive to wheat are able to tolerate it. The husks can be cooked as a cereal or used instead of rice. When the

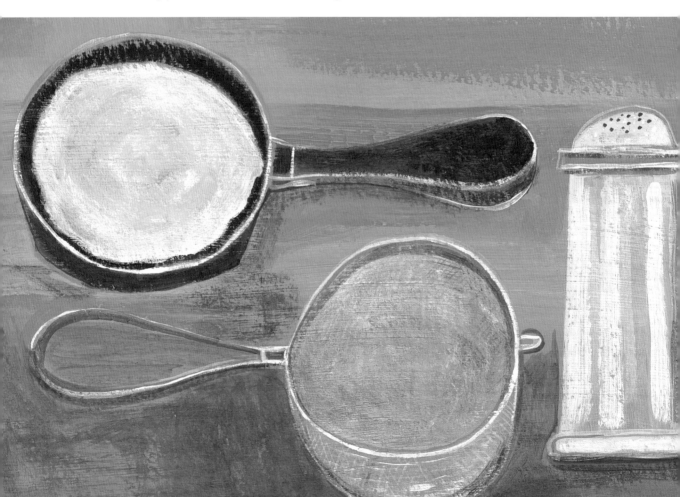

Grain	Measures of grain	Measures of water	Approximate cooking time
amaranth	1	1	20 minutes
buckwheat groats	1	2	15 minutes
millet	1	3	40 minutes
quinoa	1	2	15 minutes

groats are roasted they are called kasha. The flour tastes strong if the grain has first been roasted, but not otherwise. It can be used to make **pancakes** (see p.83) and as a substitute for wheat in baking. Buckwheat pasta, which is available commercially, is light and easily digested.

WHAT ABOUT MILLET?

Millet is useful for people who are intolerant of gluten, but as it is a grass it has to be grouped with other grasses in the rotation diet. The flavour of the whole grain, which can be used as a substitute for rice, is improved if it is toasted for a few minutes in a dry pan before being boiled. Millet flakes can be cooked like porridge or used in muesli. You may also be able to buy puffed millet as a breakfast cereal. The flour is rather grainy, like cornmeal, and can be used to make muffins or to coat meat, fish or vegetables before they are fried.

OTHER FLOURS

Gram flour made from chickpeas (garbanzo beans) can be used to make pancakes. A number of other non-grain flours, such as potato, sweet potato, sago, tapioca, water chestnut, sweet chestnut and arrowroot, can be used as thickening agents or, in certain recipes, as replacements for conventional flours.

COOKING WITHOUT EGGS

The proteins contained in eggs, even if the egg is from a different species of bird, are very similar. As a result of this you cannot usually substitute hen's eggs with those from another species. Eggs are used in cookery both to bind and thicken the ingredients, and also to add air to mixtures. Alternatives to eggs include commercial egg replacers. If you decide to use replacers always follow the instructions on the packet, and check the label to ensure they do not contain any egg or types of flour that you are excluding from your diet.

To bind mixtures, replace each egg with:

- 1tsp gelatine dissolved in 2tbsp boiling water; cool until thickened, then beat until frothy
- 2tbsp tofu: avoid if intolerant of soya beans
- 2tbsp thick fruit purée
- or substitute part of the liquid in the mixture with 25g (1oz) linseeds (flaxseeds) boiled in 250ml (8fl oz) water for 15 minutes and then cooled

As an alternative raising agent use 1tsp starch-free baking powder or 1tsp vinegar (if allowed) per egg being replaced.

69

The Candida diet

If you think that you have problems with Candida (see p.44), you should first follow the mini-elimination diet stage 1 (see p.58). For many people further dietary changes are unnecessary, but you may have to continue the diet for up to three months.

FOODS CONTAINING YEASTS AND MOULDS

- **Bread**, including pitta bread, sourdough and pizzas. Soda bread is usually yeast free, but check the label as yeast may be a secondary raising agent; in addition,

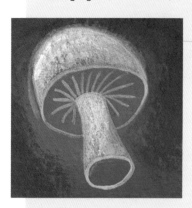

some people are sensitive to soured milk. Yeasted buns and cakes e.g. doughnuts and Danish pastries.
- **Yeast extract** and most stock cubes.
- **Anything containing 'hydrolyzed vegetable protein', or 'leavening'.**

- **Beer, wine, cider** and, to a lesser extent, whisky, brandy and other spirits.
- **Vinegar** (except spirit vinegar) and pickles (use fresh lemon juice in salad dressings).
- **Sauerkraut**
- **Vitamin supplements** unless 'yeast free'.
- **Fruit that is dried, over ripe or unpeeled**, and also olives, melons (fresh or dried), desiccated coconut, peanuts and peanut products as these are all prone to mould. Nuts should be freshly shelled if possible; or buy from a shop with a good turn-over and keep frozen.
- **Commercial fruit juices**
- **Foods containing 'malt'**
- **Synthetic cream**, fermented dairy products.
- **Smoked foods**
- **Soy sauce**, shoyu, etc.

Check labels of other sauces that may contain fermented products.
- **Leftover food** stored at room temperature for more than 24 hours, or more than 48 hours in a refrigerator (use your freezer instead).
- **Mushrooms** and other edible fungi.
- **Quorn** and mycoprotein.
- **Blue cheese**, and ripe cheeses such as Brie and Camembert.
- **Dry herbs** may contain mould, so use fresh whenever possible.

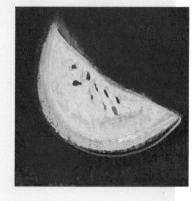

If, after 4–6 weeks of following the mini-elimination diet stage 1, you have failed to make sufficiently good progress, you should make the additional following dietary changes:

- **Check that you are still rigorously avoiding refined sugar** (see p.57).
- **Exclude all yeasts and moulds** (see p.70). Although you may be able to tolerate some of these foods, it is difficult to know which at this stage. (See also p.27.)
- **Check that you are not eating any refined-carbohydrate foods** (see p.108), and avoid eating too many whole grain carbohydrates. To avoid hunger, you may need to eat more lean meat, fish, green leafy vegetables and unsweetened natural live yogurt.
- **Limit your fresh fruit intake** to two fruits a day, and avoid those that are very sweet or over-ripe. Eat 3–6 portions of fresh vegetables each day (see p.108). Small amounts of fruit juice, freshly prepared and diluted with the same volume of water, may be taken as an occasional treat.

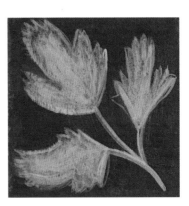

- **Unless you are infusing fresh herbs, limit herbal tea** intake to a maximum of 2–3 cups a day, as all dried herbs are to some extent mouldy. Drink at least 8 glasses of water a day; hot water can be very comforting, especially in cold weather.
- **Avoid drinking large amounts of milk**, as milk (but not yogurt) contains a sugar, lactose. You only need to exclude milk completely if you are intolerant of it.
- **Consider starting a course of prebiotics and probiotics** (see p.112) if you are not already taking them.

WHAT TO DO NEXT

Assess your symptoms after three months. How are you feeling?

Very much better: start testing your reaction to individual foods containing yeasts and moulds (see pp.98–101). You can reintroduce some sugar, but you may have a relapse if you overdo it.

Better but still not well: continue with the diet for another three months, as progress can be slow. If you are still not better then, you may have food intolerance, so progress to the mini-elimination diet plan stage 2 (p.60).

Very little progress: Candida/dysbiosis is unlikely to be a problem, so you should see your doctor as you may have an unrelated condition. If not, start the mini-elimination diet plan stage 2 (p.60), as you may have food intolerance.

pp.98-101

p.60

p.60

Non-allergic food reactions

Even plants that have been used for medicinal purposes for thousands of years can cause a reaction that can be similar to the symptoms of allergies. Some of the plants we eat as food have similar effects as well.

SALICYLATES

Although aspirin is now manufactured, it was originally extracted from willow trees. Many other plants, including those that we eat as food, contain very similar substances, known as salicylates. In susceptible people, these substances can cause **urticaria** (p.20), **rhinitis** and nasal polyps (see pp.28–9), and **asthma** (see p.30).

To test your reaction to salicylates, exclude foods high in salicylates (see box) for two weeks, and avoid aspirin and related non-steroidal anti-inflammatory medicines (check with your doctor if these are prescribed). After the two weeks eat generous portions of foods high in salicylates and monitor your symptoms. These may take a few days to develop, as the effect is cumulative. If symptoms recur or worsen, you will probably be able to control them by limiting your intake of the listed foods. If not consult a dietitian.

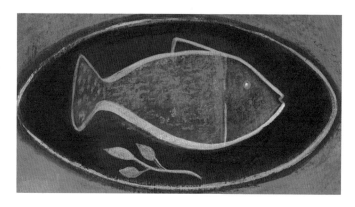

HIGH-SALICYLATE FOODS

- **Herbs and spices:** dill, tarragon, rosemary, sage, thyme, oregano and mixed herbs, aniseed, cayenne, celery powder, cinnamon, curry powder, Chinese five spices, mace, mustard, turmeric, allspice, bayleaf, chilli, cloves, ginger, mint, nutmeg, black pepper, pickles.
- **Fruit and nuts:** raisins, prunes, sharp apples, berries, citrus fruits, currants and other dried fruits, figs, guavas, grapes, kiwis, pineapples, almonds, pistachios, macadamias, pine nuts.
- **Vegetables:** broccoli, chicory, endive, gherkin, mushroom, peppers (bell peppers), radish, watercress.
- **Other:** honey, liquorice, peppermint, chewing gum, tea, rum, port, Benedictine, Tia Maria, Drambuie.
- **Salicylates are also present in:** toothpaste, antiseptic lozenges and mouthwashes, painkillers, cold cures and cosmetics. Your pharmacist will be able to guide you. If you are sensitive to aspirin, you should inform your dentist as well as your doctor, as dentists sometimes use aspirin wicks.

Foods that are low in salicylates can be eaten freely at any time. These include:

- **All kinds of meat and fish**
- **Milk, cheese and eggs**
- **Wheat, rye, barley and rice**
- **Fruit:** banana, peeled pear, lemon, pomegranate, papaya, passion fruit, mango
- **Vegetables:** cabbage, Brussels sprouts, bean sprouts, celery, leeks, lettuce, peas, peeled potatoes
- **Alcoholic drinks:** gin and vodka
- **Carob, cocoa, cashew nuts**

HISTAMINE AND RELATED SUBSTANCES

In one type of allergic reaction, histamine is released from the **mast cells** in the body (see p.21). Similar symptoms can be produced when you eat foods that either contain histamine (fermented cheeses, sausages, tinned fish, sauerkraut and spinach) or cause it to be released in the body (egg white, shellfish, tomato, chocolate, pork, pineapple, strawberry, papaya and alcohol). This is often known as a 'false food allergy'. Susceptibility to false food allergy appears to be increased in people who are **deficient in magnesium** (see p.113). Avoiding these foods may control your symptoms, which include:

- A flare-up of **eczema** (p.16), or **urticaria** (p.20)
- **Hot flushes**
- **Angioedema** (see p.20)
- **Thirst, nausea and diarrhoea**
- **Migraine** (see p.40)

Other foods contain similar substances, chemically known as amines. These can cause migraine headaches because they cause **blood vessels to dilate** (see p.40). The foods concerned include chocolate, cheese, fermented foods such as alcohol, yeast extract, pickled herrings, bananas, broad beans, liver and some sausages.

LECTINS

Lectins are substances present in a number of foods, especially dried beans. They can cause abdominal pain, diarrhoea and vomiting, but this is a toxic reaction not an allergy. Fortunately, lectins are destroyed when the beans are soaked for several hours and then boiled vigorously in an open pan for 10 minutes before being cooked slowly until soft.

CAFFEINE

Caffeine should be regarded as a drug which can cause a number of symptoms that can be confused with allergic reactions including:

- **Insomnia, anxiety, tremor**, irritability, palpitations, sweats, restless legs
- **Lethargy**, drowsiness, depression
- **Abdominal pain**, nausea, vomiting
- **A runny nose**

Caffeine can be addictive and sudden withdrawal causes symptoms such as craving, headaches, nausea and drowsiness. It is best to allow yourself a couple of weeks to withdraw from caffeine gradually. For a list of **foods that contain caffeine** see p.59.

73

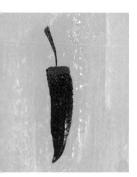

The rotation diet

A rotation diet involves eating any member of a particular food family for one or two days, and then excluding that family completely for several days. If you find you are intolerant of one member of a food family, it is quite possible that you may cross-react to another member of the same family. Occasionally, completely unrelated foods can also cross-react in the same way (see p.130). A great advantage of this diet is that it encourages you to eat a wide variety of foods.

If you follow the 8-day rotation diet suggested here, you will find that a food family eaten on days 1 and 2 is not repeated until days 9 and 10 when the rotation is started again. This regime has been chosen in order to simplify shopping and cooking. Try to choose different family members each time round. This can be difficult as far as grains are concerned, since many of the ones we eat most often belong to the grass family, which is allowed on only two days each cycle. Other starch foods are available for the days in between. Not many convenience foods fit this diet, but you can reduce the amount of time you spend in the kitchen by bulk cooking and freezing the extra food for future use.

HOW WILL A ROTATION DIET HELP?

One advantage of the rotation diet is that it makes you eat a wide range of foods. The foods that cause the most symptoms of food intolerance are those normally eaten every day, such as wheat. In the hurry of modern life, it is all too easy to fall into the habit of eating cereal for breakfast, a sandwich at midday, pasta in the evening, with biscuits in between as snacks, all of

which are wheat-based. By eating the culprit foods less frequently, the body becomes able to tolerate them. In addition, the rotation diet lowers the risk of your developing an intolerance to other foods. The immune system is also likely to benefit from the greater range of nutrients available to it.

You may well find that the rotation diet is more effective than the mini-elimination diet in identifying the foods that cause you problems. This is because eliminating a food for six days often **heightens your sensitivity** towards it (see p.96), so your symptoms become more obvious when you eat it again.

Make sure you continue with your **food, mood and symptom diary** (see p.54), and exclude any food that produces symptoms each time you eat it. Excluding the food for a few months usually allows its reintroduction without any recurrence of symptoms, but if symptoms do recur, exclude the food for a further 3–4 months before trying to reintroduce it again. The symptoms almost always disappear eventually, and then you can safely eat it once a week, twice at most.

PLANNING YOUR DIET

For each day of the diet, choose at least one helping of a protein food from an animal source, or, if you prefer, a combination of two **vegetarian proteins** (see p.57 for a list of foods). In addition, eat one or more portions of a carbohydrate food, and at least five 100g (3½oz) portions of fresh fruit and vegetables per day.

When you start your rotation diet, eliminate any foods that you are certain are causing your symptoms. Having followed the diet for a few weeks, reintroduce each of these foods (see pp.98–101), every other rotation of the diet at first, for one day. If they fail to produce symptoms, you can increase the frequency.

IF YOU DISLIKE THE FOODS SUGGESTED ON A PARTICULAR DAY

If you find the suggested rotation (see pp.82–90) leaves you with days when you dislike most of the foods, refer to the list of food families (see pp.76–9). You will find a number of foods that are the only food listed in that botanical family. This is because these foods have no close relatives that are eaten on a regular basis. These foods can easily be moved to different days of the rotation. However, if you experiment with new foods, or cook those you disliked as a child in new ways, you may find that you come to like them after all.

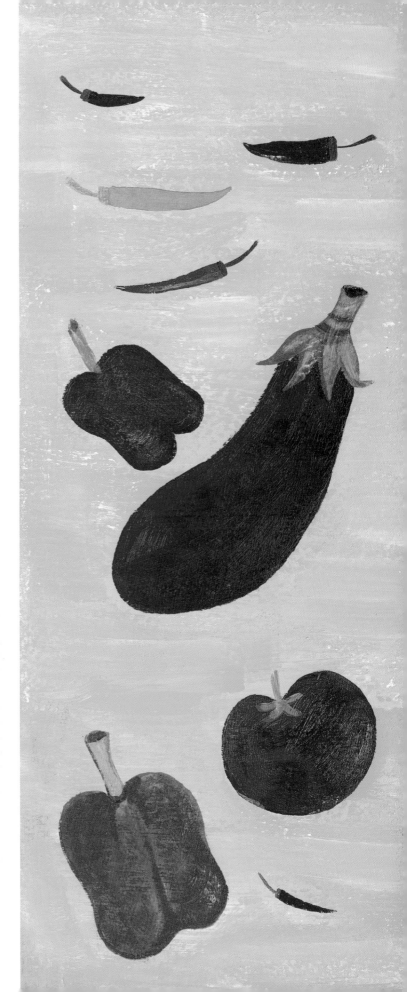

The food families

Taking rest days from the food families that cause you problems can control the symptoms of a food intolerance without your having to completely exclude too many foods from your diet. However, a very restricted diet may cause deficiency in vital nutrients. The colours allocated to the food families indicate the days of the rotation diet on which they are eaten. Purple is for days 1 and 2, green for days 3 and 4, orange for days 5 and 6, blue for days 7 and 8.

HEATH FAMILY
bilberry
blueberry
cranberry

FLAX FAMILY
linseed (flaxseed)

POULTRY FAMILY
chicken
duck
eggs (all)
goose
grouse
partridge
pheasant
pigeon
quail
turkey

BEECH FAMILY
chestnut

PEPPER FAMILY
black pepper
white pepper

PINEAPPLE FAMILY
pineapple

FUNGUS FAMILY
baker's yeast
brewer's yeast
mushroom
puffball
truffle

ARROWROOT FAMILY
arrowroot

CASHEW FAMILY
cashew
mango
pistachio

BANANA FAMILY
banana
plantain

CITRUS FAMILY
clementine
grapefruit
kumquat
lemon
lime
orange
satsuma
tangelo
tangerine
ugli fruit

GINGER FAMILY
cardamom
ginger
turmeric

BEET FAMILY
amaranth
beetroot
quinoa
spinach
sugar beet
Swiss chard

BEEF FAMILY
beef
buffalo
gelatine
goat
lamb
veal
all dairy products including:
  butter
  cheese
  milk
  yogurt

POPPY FAMILY
poppy seed

GRAPE FAMILY

- cream of tartar
- currant
- grape
- grapeseed
- raisin
- sultana

BRASSICA FAMILY

- broccoli
- Brussels sprouts
- cabbage
- cauliflower
- Chinese leaves
- cress
- horseradish
- kale
- kohlrabi
- mustard
- mustard seed
- radish
- rapeseed (canola)
- swede (rutabaga)
- turnip
- watercress

BIRCH FAMILY

- hazelnut

BUCKWHEAT FAMILY

- buckwheat
- rhubarb
- sorrel

CAPER FAMILY

- caper

DAISY FAMILY

- camomile
- chicory
- dandelion
- endive
- globe artichoke
- Jerusalem artichoke
- lettuce
- romaine lettuce
- safflower
- salsify
- steria (sweetener)
- sunflower
- tarragon

CARROT FAMILY

- anise
- caraway
- carrot
- celeriac
- celery
- chervil
- coriander (cilantro)
- cumin
- dill
- fennel
- parsley
- parsnip

MALLOW FAMILY

- okra

CONIFER FAMILY

- juniper berry
- pine nuts

FISH FAMILY (Bony*)

- anchovy
- bass
- cod
- haddock
- hake
- halibut
- herring
- mackerel
- mullet
- pilchard
- plaice
- salmon
- sardine
- sea bass
- sea bream
- sole
- trout
- tuna
- turbot
- whitebait

*Many people who are sensitive to fish are in fact reacting to a particular protein. This protein is found in bony fish, but may not be present in cartilaginous fish.

FISH FAMILY (Cartilaginous)

- dogfish
- ray
- shark
- skate

NUTMEG FAMILY

- mace
- nutmeg

THE DIET PLAN

GRASS FAMILY
bamboo shoots
barley
cane sugar
corn (maize)
kamut
lemon grass
malt
millet
oats
rice
rye
sorghum
spelt
teff
triticale
wheat
wild rice

LAUREL FAMILY
avocado
bay leaf
cinnamon

CRUSTACEAN FAMILY
crab
crayfish
lobster
prawn
shrimp

LILY FAMILY
aloe vera
asparagus
chive
garlic
leek
onion
sarsaparilla
shallot

DEER FAMILY
elk
moose
venison

DILLENIA FAMILY
kiwi fruit
passion fruit

MOLLUSC FAMILY
clam
cockle
mussel
octopus
oyster
scallop
snail
squid

MINT FAMILY
basil
marjoram
mint (all)
oregano
rosemary
sage
savory
thyme

MORNING GLORY FAMILY
sweet potato

MADDER FAMILY
coffee

MULBERRY FAMILY
breadfruit
fig
hops
mulberry

HOLLY FAMILY
maté tea

HONEYSUCKLE FAMILY
elderberry

MAPLE FAMILY
maple syrup

MELON FAMILY
courgette (zucchini)
cucumber
gherkin
marrow
melons (all) including:
  cantaloupe
  honeydew
  watermelon
pumpkins (all)
squashes (all)

NIGHTSHADE FAMILY
aubergine (eggplant)
cayenne
chilli
paprika
pepper (bell pepper)
potato
tobacco
tomato

OLIVE FAMILY
black olive
green olive

ORCHID FAMILY
vanilla

PALM FAMILY
coconut
date
sago

PEDALIUM FAMILY

sesame

PROTEA FAMILY

macadamia nuts

SAPUCAYA

brazil nut

ROSE FAMILY

almond
apple
apricot
blackberry
cherry
crab apple
damson
dewberry
loganberry
loquat
nectarine
peach
pear
pectin
plum
prune
quince
raspberry
rose hip
sloe
strawberry

SAXIFRAGE FAMILY

currants (red, white and black)
gooseberry

MYRTLE FAMILY

allspice
clove
guava

PEA FAMILY

alfalfa
beans (all) including:
 broad beans
 french (green) beans
 runner beans
dried beans (all) including:
 aduki beans
 black beans
 black-eyed beans
 butter beans
 cannellini beans
 flageolet beans
 haricot beans
 kidney beans
 lima beans
 mung beans
 pinto beans
 soya beans
carob
fenugreek
lentils (all) including:
 puy lentil
 red lentil
 green lentil
liquorice
peanuts (groundnuts)
peas (all) including:
 chickpeas (garbanzo beans)
 dried peas
 mangetout
 split-green peas
 split-yellow peas
 sugar peas
tofu

RABBIT FAMILY

hare
rabbit

SEAWEED FAMILY

agar-agar
arame
carrageen
dulse
kelp
kombu
nori
wakame

STERCULLIA FAMILY

cocoa

SEDGE FAMILY

water chestnut

SOAPBERRY FAMILY

lychee

SPURGE FAMILY

cassava
tapioca

WALNUT FAMILY

butternut
hickory nut
pecan
walnut

YAM FAMILY

yam

SWINE FAMILY

pork
wild boar

PAPAYA FAMILY

papaya

TEA FAMILY

green tea, black tea

The rotation diet chart

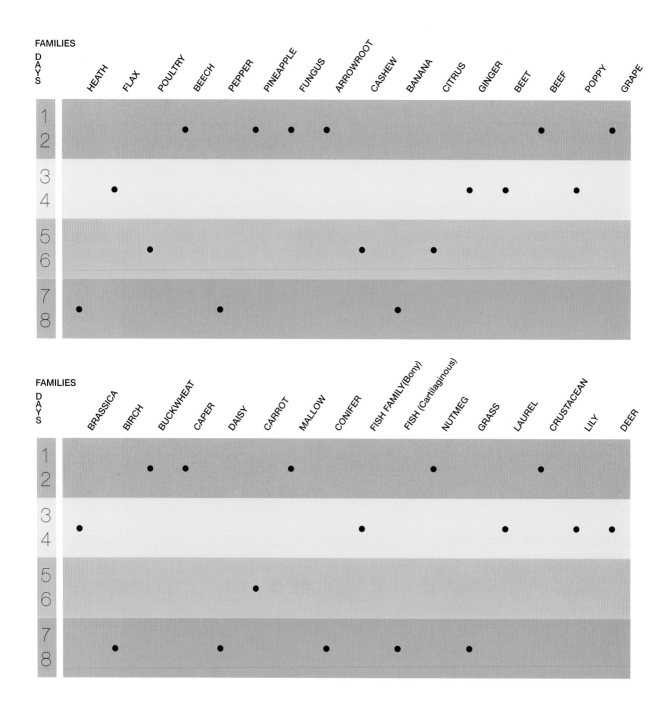

THE ROTATION DIET CHART

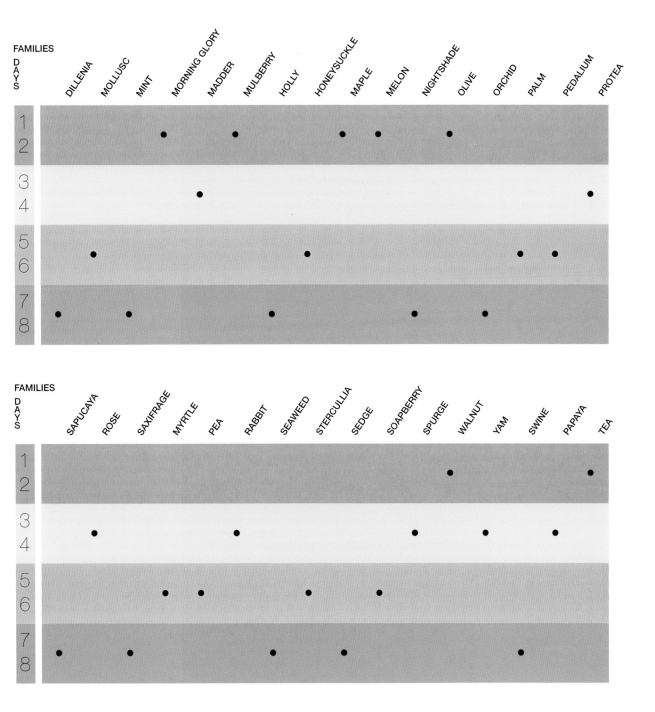

The rotation diet
DAYS 1 AND 2

Protein: cheese; milk; yogurt; beef; buffalo; goat; lamb; veal; crab; crayfish; lobster; prawn; shrimp.

Vegetables: mushrooms; puffballs; truffles; sweet potato; cucumber; breadfruit; okra; sorrel gherkins; marrow; all pumpkins and squashes; courgettes (zucchini).

Fruit: all melons, including cantaloupe, honeydew, watermelon; currants; grapes; raisins; sultanas; black olives; green olives; figs; hops; mulberries; pineapple; rhubarb.

Grains, seeds and nuts: pumpkin seeds; butternuts; hickory nuts; pecans; walnuts; chestnuts; buckwheat.

Sweeteners: maple syrup.

Fat/oil: grapeseed oil; dripping from meat; butter; olive oil.

Herbs and spices: mace; nutmeg; capers.

Drinks: milk; green and black tea; juices from fruits and milk from nuts of the day.

Miscellaneous: gelatine, baker's yeast, brewer's yeast, cream of tartar, arrowroot, yeast extract.

BUTTERNUT SOUP

1kg (2¼lb) butternut squash
3 medium courgettes (zucchini)
25g (1oz) butter
1 heaped tsp ground nutmeg
small piece (or ½tsp ground) mace
1 litre (1¾ pints) water
sea salt
55g (2oz) soft goat's cheese, in a piece

SERVES 4

Seed, peel and cube the squash, and peel and slice the courgettes. Heat the butter in a deep pan and add the nutmeg and mace. Cook for 1–2 minutes, then add the vegetables. Cover the pan and sweat on a very low heat for 15 minutes. Add the water, seasoning well, and bring to the boil and simmer for 20–30 minutes or till the squash is quite soft. Purée the soup in either a blender or food processor, then return to the pan. Bring back to the boil and simmer for a further 15 minutes to intensify the flavour, then adjust the seasoning to taste. Cut the goat's cheese into matchsticks. Pour the soup into four bowls and gently swirl some cheese into each before serving.

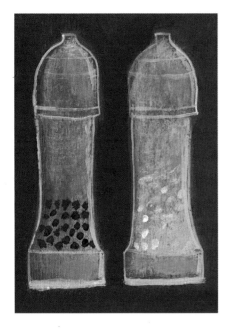

MENU SUGGESTIONS

Breakfast	Minute steak with sautéed mushrooms.
	Buckwheat pancakes (see below) and maple syrup.
Light meal	Butternut soup (see opposite) and buckwheat crispbread (see p.63).
	Baked sweet potato and grated cheese.
Main meal	Lamb chops with courgettes and steamed pumpkin.
	Paella made with kasha (see p.69).
Dessert	Stewed rhubarb with maple syrup and cream.

BUCKWHEAT PANCAKES

85g (3oz) buckwheat flour
200ml (7fl oz) water
4tbsp olive oil
50g (1 ¼lb) mixed wild
  and cultivated
  mushrooms, wiped
85g (3oz) pecan nuts,
  quartered
85g (3oz) walnuts, quartered
sea salt and freshly
  ground black pepper
4tsp plain, live yogurt,
  preferably goat's or ewe's,
  as the flavour is sharper

SERVES 4

To make the pancakes: whizz the flour and water in a food processor for 2–3 minutes, then allow the mixture to stand for 10–15 minutes. Wipe a pancake pan with a small amount of the oil and heat until it begins to smoke. Pour a little of the mixture into the pan, tipping it to ensure you get a thin and even coating, and brown quickly on both sides. Repeat so you have eight pancakes – two per person. Set aside, layering the pancakes with clingfilm or greaseproof (wax) paper, and keep warm.

To make the stuffing: halve, quarter or slice the mushrooms so they are all roughly the same size. Heat the remaining olive oil in a shallow pan and cook the nuts briskly for 1–2 minutes. Add the mushrooms and continue to cook briskly until they have wilted and released their juice. Season to taste with salt and pepper. Place a spoonful of mushroom and nut filling on each pancake, roll it up and serve at once with a spoonful of yogurt drizzled over the top.

The rotation diet
DAYS 3 AND 4

LEEK SALAD

1 large or 2 small leeks, trimmed and
   very finely sliced
200g (7oz) Chinese leaves, thinly sliced
1 bunch watercress, roughly chopped
25g (1oz) whole almonds
25g (1oz) macadamia nuts, halved
1 large sharp eating (dessert) apple,
   cored
2 ripe avocados

For the dressing:
4tbsp rapeseed (canola) oil
2tbsp cider vinegar
1tsp poppy seeds
sea salt

SERVES 4

Mix together the leeks, Chinese
leaves, watercress and nuts, and
place in a salad bowl. Cut the apple
into small pieces and add to the
salad. Peel and stone the avocados,
cut them into thick slices and
spread over the top of the salad.

Mix together the ingredients for the
dressing, drizzle over the salad,
making sure the avocado pieces are
well coated. Serve at once.

Protein: rabbit; hare; elk; moose; venison; bass; trout; anchovy; cod; haddock; hake; halibut; herring; mackerel; mullet; pilchard; plaice; salmon; sardine; sea bass; sea bream; sole; tuna; turbot; whitebait.

Vegetables: broccoli; Brussels sprouts; cabbage; cauliflower; Chinese leaves; cress; kale; kohlrabi; radish; swede (rutabaga); turnip; watercress; beetroot; spinach; Swiss chard; aloe vera; asparagus; leek; onion; yam; shallot.

Fruit: apple; apricot; blackberry; crab apple; cherry; damson; dewberry; loganberry; loquat; nectarine; peach; pear; plum; prune; quince; raspberry; rose hip; sloe; strawberry; avocado; papaya.

Grains, seeds and nuts: quinoa; amaranth; macadamia nuts; almonds; poppy seeds; mustard seeds.

Sweeteners: beet sugar.

Fat/oil: rapeseed (canola); linseed (flaxseed).

Herbs and spices: aloe vera; chive; garlic; sarsaparilla; cardamom; ginger; turmeric; bay leaf; cinnamon; horseradish; mustard.

Drink: coffee, juice from fruits and milk from nuts of the day.

Miscellaneous: tapioca, cassava.

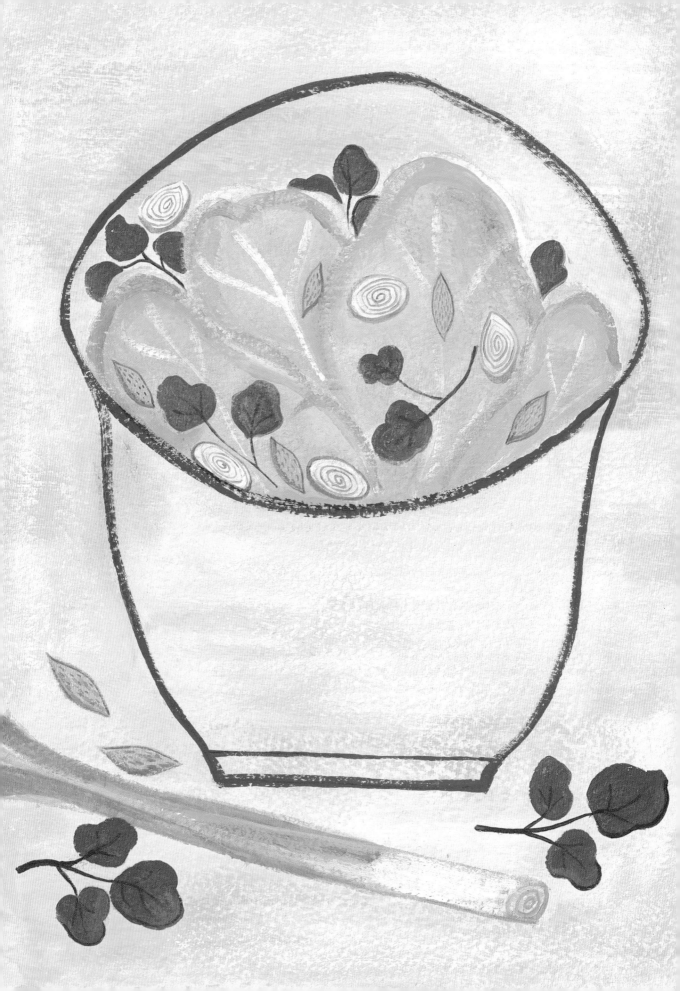

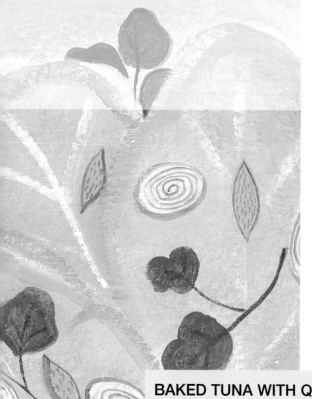

MENU SUGGESTIONS

Breakfast Quinoa porridge (see pp.68–9) with almond milk (see p.61).
     Grilled herring with tapioca crispbread (see p.63).
Light meal Grilled sardine on spinach, with cauliflower Leek salad (see p.84).
Main meal Venison stew with broccoli and baked yam.
     Baked tuna with quinoa risotto (see below).
Dessert Mixed fruit salad and almond milk.

BAKED TUNA WITH QUINOA RISOTTO

4tbsp rapeseed/
 linseed oil
12 shallots, peeled and very
 finely sliced
4 large soft prunes, stoned and
 finely chopped
350g (12oz) fresh tuna
3 large or 6 small garlic cloves,
 peeled
4 sprigs watercress

For the risotto:
2tbsp rapeseed,
 flaxseed or linseed oil
1 leek, trimmed and very finely
 sliced
170g (6oz) Swiss chard,
 washed and chopped
 fairly small
75g (2 ½oz) quinoa grains
300ml (½ pint) water
salt

SERVES 4

To cook the tuna, heat the oil in a pan just large enough to hold the tuna and add the shallots and prunes. Cover and sweat for 10 minutes or until the shallots are quite soft. Cut six small slits in the tuna and insert a small garlic clove (or a halved large clove) into each. Lay the tuna over the shallots, cover the pan, and cook gently for 30 minutes or until the tuna is cooked through.

Meanwhile, heat the oil for the risotto in a separate pan and gently cook the leek for 5 minutes. Add the Swiss chard, the quinoa grains and the water, stirring well. Season lightly, bring to the boil and simmer gently for 15–20 minutes or until the water has been absorbed and the quinoa is cooked. If necessary, add a little extra liquid.

When both are cooked, remove the tuna from the pan, spoon the shallots and cooking juices into a warmed serving dish and lay the tuna on top – either in one piece or cut into four portions if you prefer. Garnish with the watercress and serve with the quinoa risotto.

The rotation diet
DAYS 5 AND 6

Protein: chicken; duck; goose; grouse; partridge; pheasant; pigeon; quail; turkey; eggs; clams; cockles; mussels; octopus; oysters; scallops; snails; squid; tofu.

Vegetables: carrot; celeriac; celery; fennel; parsnip; alfalfa; all beans, including broad beans, french beans, runner beans; all dried beans, including aduki beans, black beans, black-eyed beans, butter beans, cannellini beans, flageolet beans, haricot beans, kidney beans, lima beans, mung beans, pinto beans, soya beans; all peas, including chick-peas , dried peas, mangetout, split-green peas, split-yellow peas, sugar peas; carob; puy, red and green lentils; liquorice.

Fruit: clementine; grapefruit; kumquat; lemon; lime; orange; satsuma; tangelo; tangerine; ugli; coconut; date; elderberry; guava; lychee; mango.

Grains, seeds and nuts: cashew; pistachio; peanut (groundnut); sesame.

Sweeteners: date syrup.

Fat/oil: peanut (groundnut); soya; sesame seed.

Herbs/spices: anise; caraway; chervil; coriander; cumin; dill; fennel; parsley; fenugreek; allspice (cilantro); clove.

Drink: cocoa, carob, juices from fruits and milk from nuts of the day, fennel tea.

Miscellaneous: sago.

TOFU BAKE

2tbsp soya oil

2 heaped tsp ground cumin

1tsp coriander seeds

1 fennel bulb

3 sticks celery

55g (2oz) puy lentils

170g (6oz) red lentils

1 litre (1 ¾ pints) water

1tsp tamari or wheat-free soy sauce

140g (5oz) smoked tofu, cubed

115g (4oz) cashew nuts

115g (4oz) mangetout,
   cut into slivers

SERVES 4

Heat the oil in a heavy-based pan and add the ground cumin and coriander seeds. Chop both the fennel and celery fairly small and add to the pan. Cover and sweat for 10–15 minutes. Add both types of lentil, the water and the tamari. Bring to the boil, cover, and simmer for about 1 hour or until the red lentils are almost entirely disintegrated and most of the liquid has been absorbed. Add the tofu and the cashew nuts and continue to cook for a further 10 minutes. Add the mangetout, stir well, and cook for another minute or so to amalgamate the flavours. Taste and season further with tamari if needed. Serve with a green salad.

MENU SUGGESTIONS

Breakfast	Gram flour pancake (see below).
	Boiled egg with gram (chickpea) flour
	crispbread (see p.63).
Light meal	Turkey stir-fry with bean sprouts and
	carrots.
	Thick bean and celeriac soup.
Main meal	Tofu bake (see p.87).
	Roast chicken, with roast parsnips
	and french beans.
Dessert	Orange and date fruit salad and
	cashew nut cream.

GRAM FLOUR PANCAKES

**100g (3 ½oz) gram
(chickpea) flour
200ml (7fl oz) water
a pinch of salt**

For the filling:
**4 kumquats
4 fresh (or well
softened dried)
dates, stoned
8 fresh lychees
12 pistachio nuts
1 large mango**

SERVES 4

Mix the flour, water and salt in a processor until you have a smooth batter. Allow the mixture to stand for 10–15 minutes. Heat a pancake pan with a dribble of oil. Pour a small ladleful of the mixture into the pan and brown quickly on both sides. Repeat so that you have four pancakes – one per person. Stack the pancakes layered with a piece of clingfilm or greaseproof paper. Keep warm.

Cut the kumquats into thin slices. Chop the dates into small pieces. Shell and stone the lychees and cut in half. Shell the pistachio nuts and also cut in half. Peel and purée the mango, then mix in the fruit and nuts – it should not need any further sweetening. Using a slotted spoon, place a spoonful of the fruit and nut mixture, reserving some for later, on one half of each pancake. Fold over and lay on a serving dish. Cover and heat gently in a microwave (1–2 minutes on high). Serve with the reserved mango purée spooned over them.

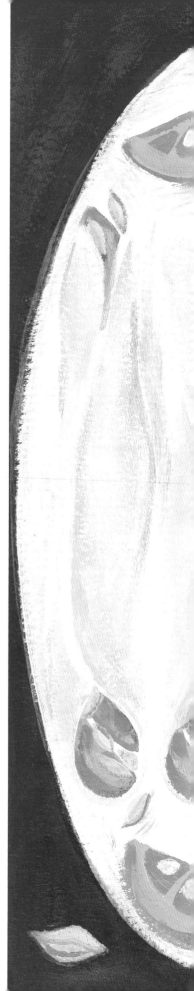

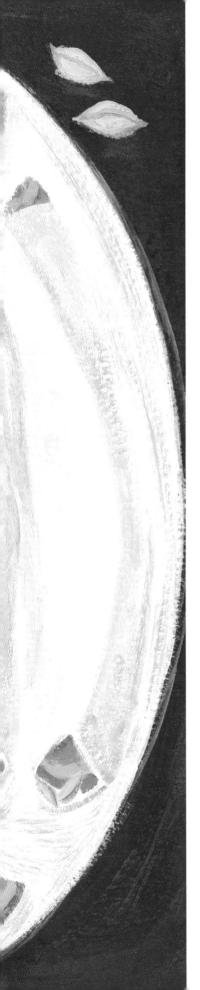

The rotation diet
DAYS 7 AND 8

Protein: pork; wild boar; shark; ray; skate; dogfish.

Vegetables: bamboo shoots; chicory; chillies; dandelion; endive; globe artichoke; Jerusalem artichoke; lettuce; romaine lettuce; salsify; aubergine (eggplant); pepper (bell pepper); potato; tomato; water chestnut; agar-agar; arame; carrageen; dulse; kelp; kombu; nori; wakame.

Fruit: blueberry; bilberry; cranberry; banana; plantain; kiwi fruit; passion fruit; red, white and black currants; gooseberry.

Grains, seeds and nuts: barley; corn (maize); kamut; millet; oats; rice; rye; sorghum; spelt; teff; triticale; wheat; wild rice; sunflower seeds; hazelnuts; brazil nuts; pine nuts.

Sweeteners: cane sugar; malt syrup; rice syrup; stevia (sweetener).

Fat/oil: corn (maize); safflower; hazelnut; sunflower.

Herbs/spices: camomile; tarragon; juniper berry; all members of the mint family – basil, marjoram, oregano, rosemary, sage, savory, thyme; vanilla; white and black pepper; paprika; chilli; lemon grass; cayenne.

Drink: maté tea; juices from fruits and milk from nuts of the day; mint tea; camomile tea; oat milk; rice milk.

Miscellaneous: tobacco (see p.46).

MENU SUGGESTIONS

Breakfast   Grilled bacon and tomato. Wheat flakes with banana and hazelnut milk.

Light meal   Baked potato and salad. Pasta with a sauce made from stewed (bell) peppers and tomato.

Main meal   Pork chop, mashed potato, braised chicory. Stir-fried pork.

Desert   Fruit mousse (see below).

FRUIT MOUSSE

4 large bananas
4 large kiwi fruit
3 large passion fruit
25g (1oz) cornflour (cornstarch)
blueberries or redcurrants to decorate

SERVES 4

Peel the bananas and kiwi fruit and put in a food processor. Halve the passion fruit, scoop out the seeds, and add to the other fruit. Purée. In a small saucepan, mix the cornflour with a couple of tablespoons of the fruit purée. Heat gently, stirring all the time, until the mixture thickens, then gradually add the rest of the purée. Pour into 4 glasses or bowls and chill. To serve, decorate with blueberries or redcurrants.

STIR-FRIED PORK

2tbsp corn (maize) oil
1 medium-sized hot chilli, seeded and finely sliced
1 green, 1 yellow and 1 red (bell) pepper, seeded and fairly finely sliced
1 large Jerusalem artichoke, trimmed, scrubbed and cut into matchsticks
2 roots of salsify, peeled and cut into matchsticks
1 medium aubergine (eggplant), diced
115g (4oz) pork fillet, cut into matchsticks
1tbsp arame, soaked for 10 minutes in water
sea salt
freshly ground black pepper
50g (2oz) sunflower seeds
25g (1oz) pine nuts

SERVES 4

Heat the oil in a wok or large frying pan with a lid until the oil begins to smoke, then add the chilli, peppers, artichoke, salsify, aubergine and pork. Stir-fry the ingredients briskly for 5–8 minutes until the vegetables start to soften, then add the arame. Season with salt and pepper, then cover, reduce the heat to low and allow to cook for a further 8–10 minutes or until the pork is cooked through. Add the sunflower seeds and pine nuts. Adjust the seasoning to taste. Serve the stir fry at once, accompanied with rice and/or a green salad.

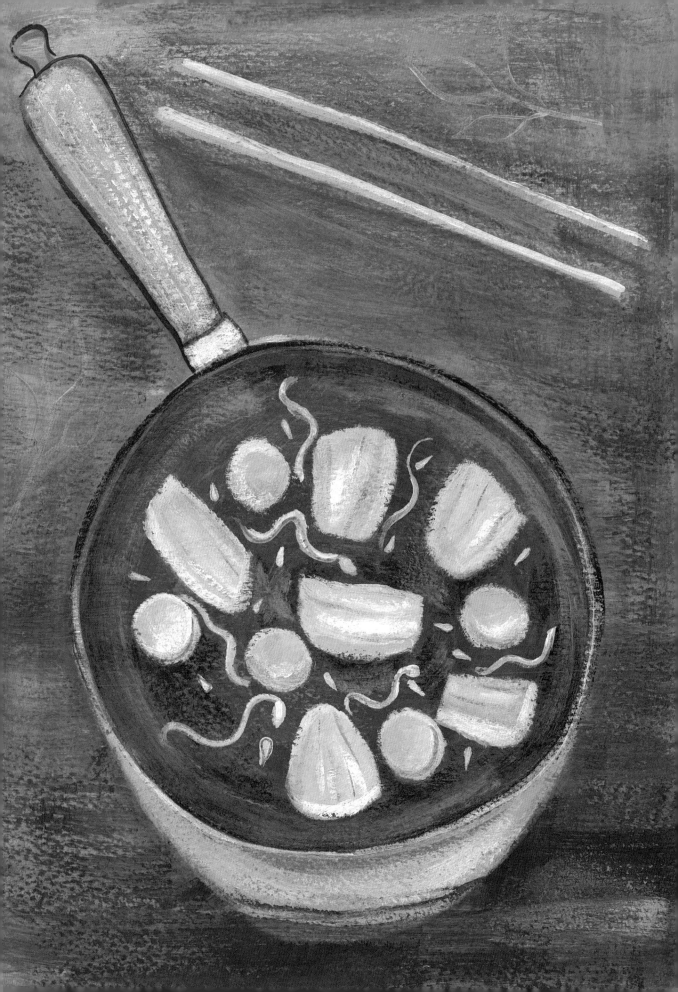

Sprouted seeds

Sprouted seeds have been eaten for many thousands of years and in many cultures. In areas such as the Himalayas, which are very cold in winter, they are an essential source of high-quality nutrients at a time of year when other fresh foods are difficult to obtain.

The seed is a storehouse of energy and nutrients needed by a young plant in its first few days of life. Many of these nutrients are stored in inactive forms, but as soon as germination starts they undergo the chemical changes which enable them to provide the seedling with essential and readily available nutrients – nutrients that can benefit us when we eat the seedling.

If you want to sprout your own seeds, it is possible to buy a commercially made sprouter, but you can get just as good results from using a glass jar.

WHAT TO DO

Place the seeds in a jar and soak them in plenty of spring or filtered water, or tap water that has been first boiled and cooled to disperse the chlorine added during purification. Pour off the water, rinse with fresh water and allow the jar to drain for a minute or so. Stretch some muslin, or similar fabric, across the opening and secure with a rubber band. Place the jar in a warm, dark place (such as an airing cupboard) for a few days, but remember to rinse the seeds 2–3 times each day. Once the seeds have sprouted, you can store any that you do not want to eat immediately in a plastic bag or box in the refrigerator for up to 5 days. Wash the jar and muslin in hot water before growing the next crop, to deter mould growth.

Seed	Soak time (hours)	When ready (days)	Notes
alfalfa	4	5–6	place in light for final day
chickpeas	18–24	3–4	can be cooked after 2 days
lentils	16	2 for salad	use whole lentils not the split red ones
		5 for juicing	
mung beans	16-24	2–3 for salad	tend to be bitter if exposed to light
		4 for juicing	
mustard	6–8	4–5	grow on damp paper, in light; cut green tops
sunflower	12	1–2	bruise easily, handle with care

WHAT TO DO NEXT

Assess your symptoms after three months. How do you feel?

About the same: Chemicals in your environment may be hampering your progress, especially if you feel better when away from home and work, or after spending more time in the fresh air. Try to **reduce your exposure to chemicals** and **continue with the diet** for 4–6 weeks (see also p.48, p.98 and pp.126–30). If your symptoms are no better, consult a doctor who is experienced in environmental medicine for personal advice and, possibly, **neutralization or EPD** (see p.137). If such a consultation is impossible, consider starting the **elimination diet** (see p.94).

Better but still not fully well: Reduce your exposure to chemicals (see above). If this does not help, try to seek advice from a doctor experienced in environmental medicine. If this isn't possible, remaining on the rotation diet for longer may help, though you may feel that the effort is too great for the improvement gained. Only you can make this decision. Alternatively, you could relax the diet, as suggested below, or consider following the **elimination diet** (p.94).

Very much better: Stay on the rotation diet until you have **reintroduced most of the foods** that have caused symptoms (see p.98). If you only react to a food sometimes, you may be able to tolerate it if it is organic. At this stage taking the occasional day off from your diet is unlikely to cause you any problems. Once you have reintroduced most foods, start to relax the rotation diet for food groups that have not caused any problems. For example, you may never have had any problems with meat or fresh produce. However, it is important that you continue to eat a wide range of different foods and rotate any food families that have previously caused symptoms. Alternatively, you may find that continuing to exclude them completely when eating at home allows you to eat freely when eating out. For many people this is the easiest and most socially acceptable way to run their lives, as being picky about food can be embarrassing; it can also make you less welcome as a guest.

pp.48, 94, 98, 126–30, 137

p.94

p.98

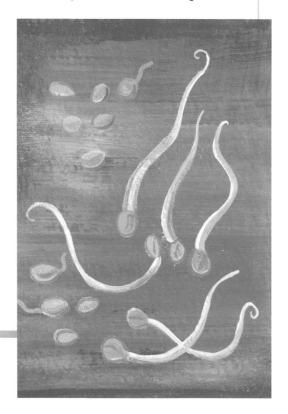

The elimination diet plan
STAGE 1

The elimination diet plan follows a very strict regime, and to achieve beneficial results, you need to keep accurate records of the foods you have excluded. Ideally, you should be under the supervision of a doctor who has some experience of caring for people undertaking this type of diet. Supervision is essential for children, vegetarians and vegans, or if you are underweight.

During stage 1, it is essential not to eat or drink anything other than what is on the list of permitted foods, so do not start the diet until it is possible for you to completely control your intake of food and drink. If you take regular medication, consult your doctor about stopping it, or switching to a brand that does not contain fillers derived from foods that are not permitted. The birth control pill contains lactose and is best stopped at the end of a cycle, and alternative contraceptive measures started immediately.

During the first week of this diet, the number of foods you can eat is strictly limited. Do not eat canned or shop-bought frozen food. Home-freezing is permitted provided you do not add ingredients that are not on the list. Unwrap any food that has been stored in plastic bags or

PREPARING FOR THE DIET

- **Buy or borrow some bathroom scales** and always use the same ones.
- **Learn to take your pulse**, which you can feel on the thumb side of your wrist; count the beats for 30 seconds and multiply by two. During stage 1, record your resting pulse rate after sitting quietly for a few minutes. As you start to reintroduce foods, changes in your pulse rate can help to pinpoint reactions (see p.98).
- **Try to reduce your exposure to chemicals**, including tobacco smoke, as much as possible (see p.48 and pp.126–30). Replace your toothpaste with bicarbonate of soda (baking soda). Avoid licking stamps and envelopes as the glue is made from corn (maize) and contains chemicals.
- **Modify your mood, food and symptom diary** (see p.54) to record your weight twice a day, and any unexpected exposure to chemicals, such as someone's perfume. When you start to reintroduce foods, you will also need to keep lists of safe foods, suspect foods and those that have definitely caused symptoms. Keep written records as this diet is far too disruptive to be undertaken more than once. Even if your memory is good, you may find that you need to refer to your records in a few months' time.

containers about two hours prior to eating or cooking, to allow plastic fumes to disperse. Avoid any food on the list that you would normally eat either daily or several times a week, or that you know causes symptoms.

Choose from the following list:
- **lamb**
- **salmon, cod, plaice, mackerel** – fresh or frozen, but not canned or smoked.
- **fresh pears, kiwi fruit or peaches**
- **avocado pears, sprouted mung beans** (see p.92), sweet potatoes, parsnips, swede (rutabaga), turnips, courgettes (zucchini), marrow.
- **sunflower, safflower or olive oil** for cooking, but only one type, and choose one that you have rarely or never used before.
- **sea salt, spring water** – in glass bottles, if possible.

HOW LONG WILL STAGE 1 LAST?

Depending on your symptoms (see below), the diet will need to be followed for 7–14 days. You will find yourself eating strange meals at strange times, such as lamb and sweet potato for breakfast. You should avoid being hungry, but do not eat or drink any item that is not on the list. The time on the diet can be shortened (unless you already have diarrhoea) by taking 2 teaspoons Epsom salts dissolved in 150ml (5fl oz) spring water the first morning.

QUICK SNACKS

- Make parsnip fries by cutting the root lengthways into quarters or eighths, then boil in water for 3–4 minutes, drain, dry on kitchen paper and fry in shallow oil.
- Thinly slice a sweet potato, then either deep-fry in your chosen oil, or place the slices in a box with a lid, add a tablespoon of oil, shake gently until they are thinly coated with oil, then spread the slices on a baking tray and bake in a hot oven 230ºC (450ºF), gas mark 8 until crisp. When cool, store in a tin for a quick snack.

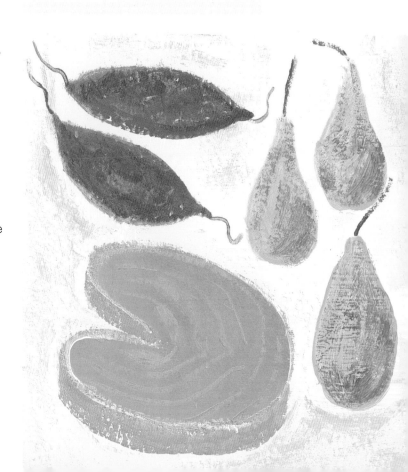

The elimination diet plan
STAGE 2

During the first few days you may feel very much worse; you may lose some weight, if you have been retaining water; and your resting pulse may become slower. These are all good signs, as they indicate that food intolerance is a problem for you. Most people feel much better by day 7 or 10 and are ready to start reintroducing foods. (If you have rheumatoid arthritis, you may need to continue stage 1 for 14 days before you feel an improvement.) However, if you find that the way you feel, or your symptoms, do not change at all, you need to seek professional advice, as it may be necessary to change the allowed foods, which requires individual advice.

Do not proceed to stage 2 unless you have noticed some changes and are beginning to feel much better. Because you have been excluding most foods for less than three weeks you will now be reintroducing foods three times a day for the first week or so, as

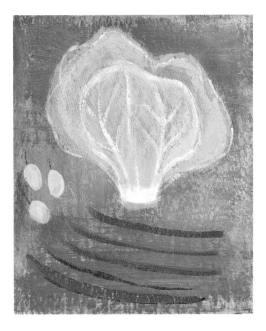

your symptoms should be more intense than they would have been after a longer break. Look out for symptoms such as headaches, joint pains, mood changes, respiratory symptoms such as a runny nose or wheezing, digestive symptoms such as diarrhoea or bloating, or any of your allergy symptoms. If you experience severe symptoms, you may find that **bicarbonate of soda (baking soda) or other mixtures** bring relief (see p.99).

All symptoms should be recorded in your **food, mood and symptom diary** (see p.54), and, at this stage, if you have a reaction, always blame the most recently reintroduced food and stop eating it immediately. Weigh yourself twice a day after emptying your bladder; if your weight increases by more than 450g (1lb) in 12 hours it is likely that you have eaten a culprit food. Add the most recently reintroduced food to your 'suspect list' and stop eating it.

Do not worry about making mistakes; you can always retest the food later (see p.98), but if you continue to eat suspect or culprit foods it will make it more difficult to work out which are the ones causing your symptoms. Reactions can vary in their intensity, and it is important not to reintroduce any more foods until your symptoms have settled down completely.

Leave at least 5 hours between meals containing a newly reintroduced food, as symptoms may not occur immediately. If there are no symptoms, you can add the new food to your list of safe foods and eat it whenever you wish, but remember that you may induce intolerance if you eat it too often. If you become hungry between meals have a snack of a safe food, and keep your diet as wide and varied as possible. This is most easily achieved by eating fresh fruit and vegetables according to their local seasons and eating a range of different grains.

Reintroduce foods in the order suggested in the box below, by eating a good-sized portion as part of your meal. The foods chosen here are the least likely to cause problems, but it is best not to reintroduce food at this stage that you have previously identified as triggering symptoms.

WHAT TO DO NEXT

You are now at the point where you can add new foods to your diet, in the same way as those people who are reintroducing foods after different stages of the Diet Plan. Follow the **general guidelines** given on pp.98–101. Since foods are reintroduced at the rate of one each day, or slightly less frequently, you may find that any reaction is less marked. It is therefore often helpful to **take your pulse**, as suggested on p.98.

pp.98–101

Day	Morning	Midday	Evening
1	banana	celery	brown rice
2	plum	carrot	turkey
3	melon	cauliflower	onion
4	grapes	cabbage	french beans
5	apple	leeks	spinach
6	parsnip	pork	broccoli

Reintroducing foods

Reintroducing excluded foods is essential, so that you can return to eating a diet that is as healthy and varied as possible. Few people with food intolerance have to exclude culprit foods indefinitely, but the foods most difficult to reintroduce are usually the ones that you should exclude first if your symptoms recur.

GENERAL GUIDANCE FOR REINTRODUCING FOODS

Modify your mood, food and symptom diary (see p.54). You should note any unexpected exposure to chemicals, such as someone's perfume, and any activity that causes symptoms, such as aching joints and muscles after a long walk. As you start to reintroduce foods, keep lists of safe foods, suspect foods and those that have definitely caused symptoms, the culprit foods.

Once you have excluded a food for more than three weeks, you may find that your symptoms, when you reintroduce it, are minimal. It is important, however, to note everything, even if you do not think it is relevant, as a pattern may emerge. A reaction can sometimes be detected by weighing yourself twice a day, either naked or wearing nightclothes, after emptying your bladder. Any gain of more than 450g (1lb) between consecutive weighings is suggestive of a reaction, unless your evening meal was eaten shortly beforehand. You may also find the pulse test helpful (see box).

Any food that does not cause a reaction can be added to the list of safe foods and eaten freely, but not too frequently. Continue to exclude any food that causes a reaction. If in doubt, leave it out, as you can always test a suspect food again later. Make a note of your symptoms and the time that they occur. When assessing your progress, you may also find that grading the symptoms by giving them marks out of ten – ten being the most severe

THE PULSE TEST

Measuring your pulse before and after eating a test food can help to pinpoint a reaction:

- Learn to take your pulse (see p.94).
- Sit quietly for five minutes before eating the food to be tested, then take your pulse and make a note of it. Eat the food and retake your pulse 20, 40 and 60 minutes later.
- You should regard the test as positive if your pulse rate alters by more than ten beats per minute. A food reaction usually increases the heart rate, but occasionally it becomes slower.
- If possible, perform the pulse test the first time you reintroduce a food. You do not need to repeat the test if it is negative. If it is positive, stop eating the food and enter it on the list of culprit or suspect foods.

you can imagine and zero being no symptoms at all – can be helpful. Symptoms may become less severe each time you test the same food.

If you have a reaction, do not test any further foods until the symptoms settle completely. To hasten relief from symptoms, you can take one of the mixtures suggested (see box). Always wait at least five days before retesting any food that you suspect may have caused a reaction.

RELIEVING SYMPTOMS OF A REACTION

Taking one of the following mixtures can usually terminate a reaction to a test food:

- 2tsp bicarbonate of soda dissolved in 150ml (5fl oz) warm water.
- 2tsp bicarbonate of soda and 1tsp potassium bicarbonate dissolved in 150ml (5fl oz) warm water. (Potassium bicarbonate can be difficult to obtain, but your local pharmacist may be able to order it for you.)
- ½–1tsp vitamin C powder with a pinch of bicarbonate of soda dissolved in 150ml (5fl oz) warm water.

If symptoms persist, you can repeat the dose once, 4–6 hours later.

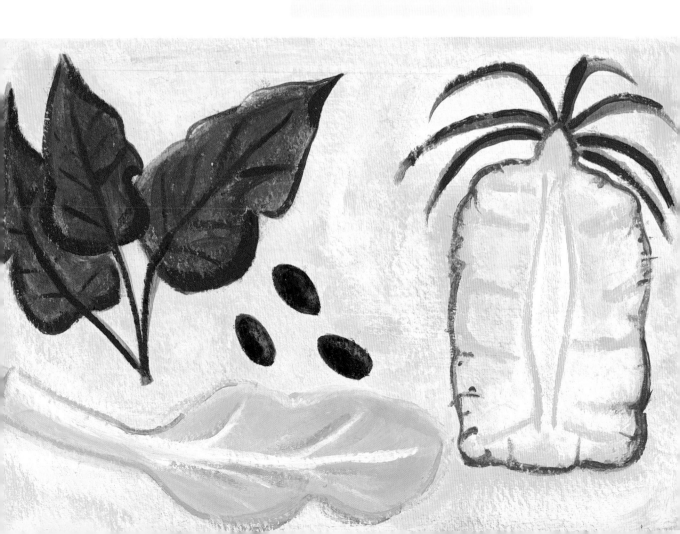

Testing the foods most frequently eaten

FOODS TO TEST FIRST

Day 1	Tap water
Day 2	Cow's milk, a glassful with each meal
Days 3, 4, 5	Wheat: eat egg-free wholemeal spaghetti or a wholewheat sugar-free cereal
	Continue for three days as symptoms may develop (and clear) slowly
Day 6	Tea: use your usual brand
Day 7	Soya* milk
Day 8	Cheddar cheese
Day 9	Beet sugar
Days 10, 11	Oats as porridge or oat cakes (check the label for added ingredients)
Day 12	Eggs: one with each meal
Day 13	Ground coffee (not instant; see box, opposite)
Day 14	Butter
Days 15, 16	Corn* (maize): have corn on the cob at each meal, plus 2tsp pure glucose powder, which is derived from corn (maize)
Day 17	Good quality plain chocolate: omit at this stage if you have reacted to corn (maize), wheat or sugar
Day 18	Mushrooms
Day 19	Peanuts (groundnuts): choose loose, additive-free nuts from a health food shop
Day 20	Cane sugar
Day 21	Oranges
Day 22	Potatoes
Day 23, 24	Rye: test with a pure rye crispbread
Day 25	Yeast: two brewer's yeast tablets three times during the day
Day 26	Malt*: mix 2tsp extract into a safe food at each meal

* Do not omit these foods even if you think you don't eat them – they are widely used in food processing and manufacture, and it is important to know whether or not they are safe for you.

Introduce new foods in the order suggested on p.100. Since it is possible to arrive at this stage from different parts of the Diet Plan the foods that are excluded will not be the same for each person. If you are already eating a test food, just go on to the following day's test. Avoid testing any food that you know or suspect to be a culprit food, as the idea at this stage is to widen your diet as rapidly as possible. Eat a reasonable portion of the test food at each meal, for one or more days as indicated, but stop if you experience a reaction and allocate the food to the **suspect or culprit lists** (see p.94). If you have no symptoms, add the food to your safe food list.

Although you will now have a reasonable choice of safe foods, this is the time to test any single-ingredient foods that have been excluded from your diet and that you are longing to eat again. If you did not react to yeast, you can even include your favourite alcoholic drink.

Before going on to eat foods with multiple ingredients you need to test your reaction to common chemicals in foods, see below:

IF YOU HAVE TO BREAK YOUR DIET...

Sometimes circumstances prevent you from adhering to your diet and you have to eat foods that are not on your permitted list. If this happens, simply return to eating the foods you know to be safe for five days. Then start the testing programme again, beginning at the stage where you left it.

TESTING FOR COMMON CHEMICALS

Day 1	White bread (provided wheat and yeast are safe). This is a test for anti-caking agents and bleaches.
Day 2	Raisins: these are treated with **sulphite preservatives** (see p.38).
Day 3	Good quality instant coffee: this contains a number of chemicals. Note that inexpensive brands often contain corn (maize).
Day 4	Canned carrots (provided you are safe with fresh carrots). A reaction suggests that you are intolerant of the resin lining the can and you will have to be careful with other canned foods.
Day 5	**Monosodium glutamate** (see p.38): sprinkle a little of this flavour enhancer over the food you are eating.
Day 6	**Artificial sweeteners:** these are often found in foods labelled 'no added sugar'. You should test them separately.
Day 7	Bacon (providing pork is safe): you are testing for **nitrites and nitrates** (see p.39)

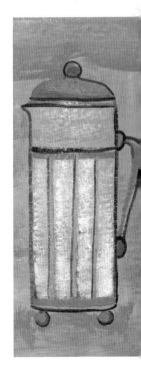

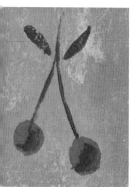

Getting back to a normal diet

Continue to add single-ingredient foods that have been excluded but that you sometimes want to eat. For clarity, add them one at a time and maintain your food, mood and symptom diary so that you can note any reactions. Then you can start to test foods with multiple ingredients, such as cakes, biscuits, jams and sauces. Read the food labels carefully, however, and avoid those that contain ingredients to which you have reacted until you know these are safe if eaten infrequently.

TROUBLESHOOTING

Determining which foods are safe can be difficult. Symptoms may return even though you have not reacted clearly to any food that you have tested. If you become confused, the following tips maybe helpful:

• Check the **food family lists** (pp.76–9) and, for a few days, remove from your diet any close relatives of foods to which you have had a strong reaction. If this does not help, return to the stage at which you last felt well and eat only safe foods for a few days before you start to test again. You may then need to retest using larger portions and allowing twice the number of days for testing. If you have not been using the **pulse test** (see p.98) you may find that it helps to identify more clearly which foods you are reacting to.

• Check how much caffeine you are taking. Even though tea, coffee and chocolate appeared not to cause reactions when they were reintroduced individually, the cumulative dose of caffeine may be producing symptoms and confusing your test results.

• You may have started to eat too many added chemicals. Retesting with organic foods can sometimes produce clearer results. Avoid eating too many manufactured and processed foods.

• You may need to obtain professional advice.

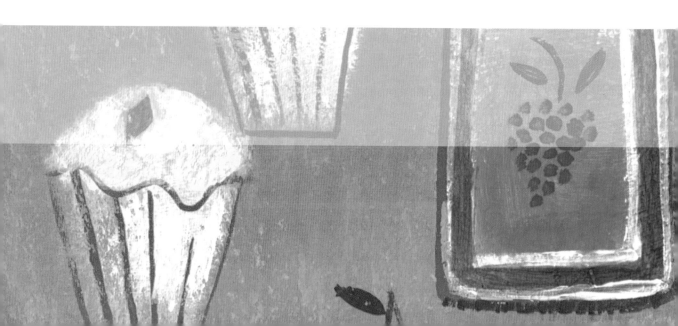

DON'T FORGET...

Anyone who is prone to food intolerance is likely to find that it is a recurring problem. If you have reached this stage, you will already have invested a lot of effort in trying to overcome it; to stay well, however, you will need to continue to be vigilant.

- **Continue to eat a diet that is as healthy and varied as you can make it** (see pp.106–13).
- **Take regular exercise** (see p.118) and practise **stress management** (see p.122) to help to maintain a healthy immune system.
- **If symptoms return, refer back to your food, mood and symptom diary** and exclude previous culprit foods for a week, then reintroduce them one at a time along the lines recommended on pp.98–101. If necessary, keep a new **food, mood and symptom diary** (see p.54) for two weeks, taking particular note of foods that you eat frequently. Exclude these for a week and then reintroduce in the same way.
- **Deal promptly with food cravings.** They either signal the emergence of a new intolerance or the return of an old one. Exclude for a week the food(s) you crave and then reintroduce it/them on a once-a-week basis.

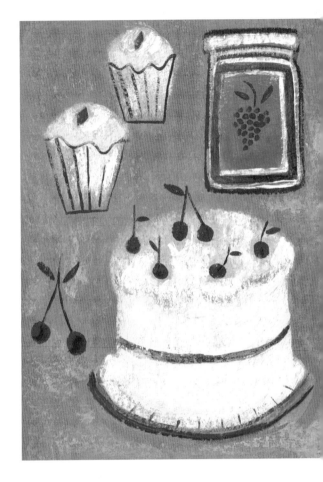

WHAT TO DO NEXT

As you should now have a list of foods that you know to be safe, you can begin retesting foods that are on your suspect list. If you find that you no longer appear to be reacting to them you can reintroduce them once or twice a week at most.

- Wait 6–12 months before reintroducing foods to which you reacted more strongly or which you excluded from your reintroduction programme because they previously caused symptoms.
- When these foods no longer appear to be causing problems, eat them occasionally. If your allergy is a seasonal one, such as hay fever, you may find that you can eat many or all of these foods freely, except during the season that your symptoms occur (see also p.130 for **cross-reactions**). If your list of problem foods is extensive, you may need to consider **neutralization, EPD** (see p.137) or **homeopathic densensitization** (see p.117).

pp.117, 130, 137

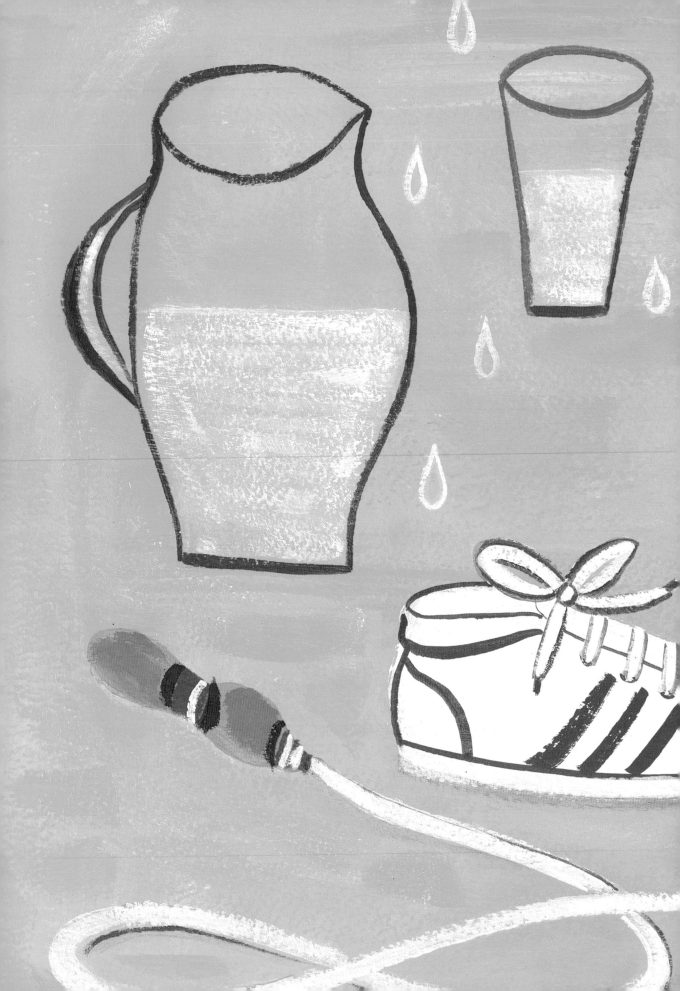

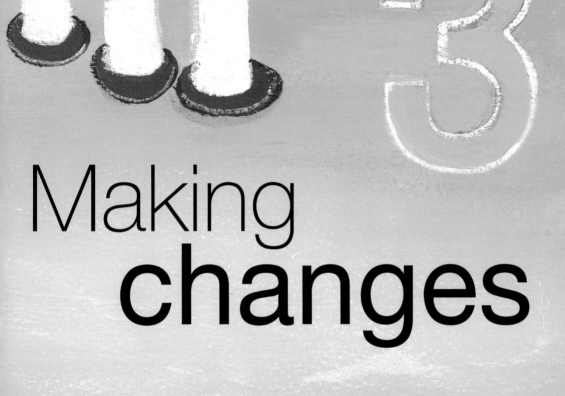

Making
changes

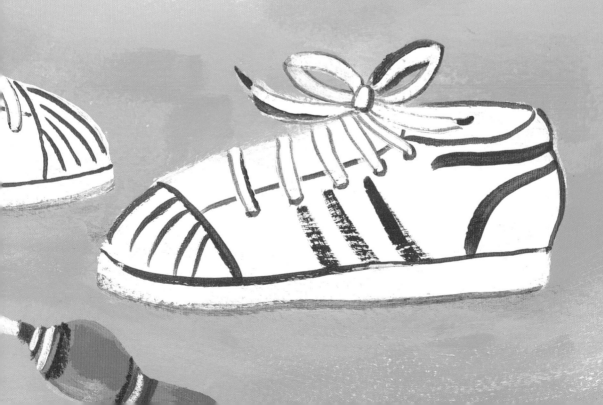

Lifestyle changes

Effective action against allergies includes keeping your immune system as healthy as possible. An initial, elementary step is to provide it with the nutrition it needs, which means eating a nutrient-rich diet and, possibly, taking nutritional and herbal supplements. Regular exercise and a reduction in your level of stress also helps, as both have been shown to improve the efficiency of the immune system.

EAT WELL TO STAY WELL

Eating well is not just a matter of consuming the right number of calories for your build and level of activity. It is much more to do with nourishing all parts of your body, including your immune system, rebuilding any worn out parts and providing a supply of energy that is available whenever it is needed.

Every day you need a supply of protein, carbohydrate and fat. Ideally, these nutrients should be present in every meal. Foods that contain them also provide the 22 minerals and 13 vitamins that are essential if certain deficiency diseases are to be avoided. In addition, scientists are discovering that there are many more beneficial compounds in fruit and vegetables than previously thought. Only by eating a wide range of different foods will you obtain enough of all these vital nutrients.

WATER TO SUSTAIN LIFE

If you do not eat you will eventually die, but if you do not drink you will die very much sooner, because water plays such a vital part in every function within the body. Every day you should be drinking between six and eight large glasses of water. If you want, you can flavour it with a little fruit juice or fruit slices.

Other healthy drinks include herbal and fruit teas, and coffee substitutes made from dandelion root, chicory, barley or rye. Normal tea and coffee, cola drinks and alcohol can be drunk in limited quantities, but they all increase the amount of urine that you pass and so contribute to dehydration, which can give you headaches, dizziness, brain fog, fatigue, dry skin and constipation, and also increase the risk of developing infections.

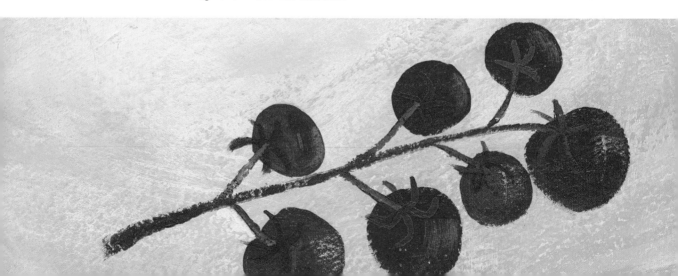

Protein for body maintenance

Protein is needed for building and repairing the different parts of the immune system, the tissues of the body and many of the chemical messengers, hormones and enzymes that are needed to maintain health and normal functions of the body.

Amino acids are the building blocks from which proteins are constructed. We obtain all the amino acids we need when we eat protein from animal sources, such as meat, fish, eggs and dairy products. Plants provide a more limited range of amino acids, as most plant protein is stored in the seeds, nuts and grains destined to grow into the next generation. To obtain the full range of amino acids from vegetable sources alone, it is necessary to eat more than one type of plant protein. Plant proteins are not, however, second class, as was once thought. They come as a health-giving package containing **fibre** (see p.109) and **essential fatty acids** (see p.110), and so should be part of every diet.

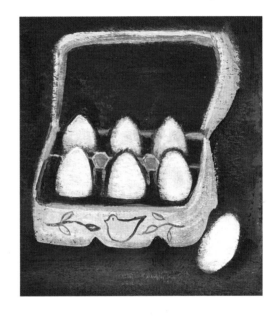

Judging how much protein to eat and getting the right balance between protein and carbohydrates is not easy. A large piece of meat or fish with a small helping of vegetables may provide too much protein and too few of the vitamins found in fruit and vegetables. A main meal consisting of white pasta with a tomato sauce will contain too little protein and lack essential amino acids. To make matters worse, both these meals contain an imbalance between the amount of protein and the amount of carbohydrate. In some people, this can cause instability in the levels of sugar in the blood, which can affect the supply of energy and lead to sugar craving. Too much sugar prevents the immune system from working properly.

A good balance between proteins and carbohydrates can be achieved by eating a reasonable portion of low-fat protein, such as meat, fish, eggs or dairy products, together with a generous helping of non-starchy **vegetables** and **fruit** (see p.108). If you want to eat more starchy foods, go for those that include the natural fibre, such as jacket potatoes and whole grains, have a smallish helping and balance it with approximately the same-sized helping of a protein food, plus plenty of non-starchy vegetables and fruit.

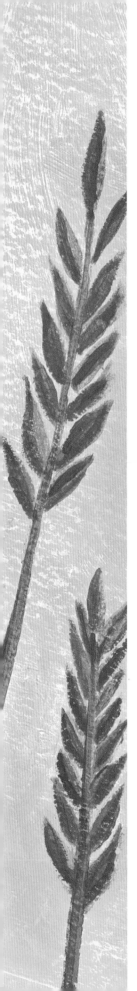

Carbohydrates and energy

Plants use energy from the sun to combine carbon dioxide with water to make carbohydrates or 'carbs', which release energy in our bodies when, after they are eaten, they are changed back into their original components. Chemically, carbohydrates are various types of sugar. Most vegetables and juicy fruits are good sources of these sugars because the sugars are diluted by the presence of water. In addition, they are good sources of minerals and vitamins and, because they are not high in calories, they can be eaten in large amounts.

When a plant stores energy for future use, such as in a potato tuber or a grain of wheat, it joins the sugar molecules together to form long molecules of starch. Starch is a concentrated form of energy, but the body has to turn it back into sugar before it can be used, so starchy foods release energy gradually over several hours. Starchy foods stave off hunger between meals, but they are concentrated sources of energy so should be eaten in moderate amounts.

When carbohydrates are eaten as whole foods, they contain plenty of **fibre** (see box, p.109), which slows down the release of sugar into the bloodstream. They are also naturally rich in minerals and vitamins, which are lost when foods are processed into white sugar and flour. Eating excessive amounts of refined sugar and white flour can upset the body's ability to control the level of sugar in the blood, causing a condition called insulin resistance, in which the level remains too high. This can both damage the tissues of the body, and reduce the effectiveness of the immune system.

HIDDEN SUGAR

The desire for sweet food seems to be inbuilt in humans, which was beneficial when feasting on sweet autumn fruits was needed to build up fat for the lean days of winter. Today, with easy access to refined sugar every day, many people are addicted to it. Manufacturers know this, and add sugar to almost all breakfast cereals, as well as savoury foods, such as soups and potato crisps. In foods promoted as being low in fat, it is often sugar that replaces the fat. Try to limit your intake of sugar to about 55g (2oz) a day. This may sound a lot, but, if you read food labels, you will find that it is very easily exceeded. On average, we eat around three times that amount each day.

Artificial sweeteners are not the answer. They make no contribution to retraining the taste

RAINBOW DIET

Mix your own phytochemicals by choosing different red, yellow, purple, brown and green fruit and vegetables on a regular basis. You can also add a glass of red wine and enjoy a piece of chocolate with 70 per cent cocoa!

buds and stopping sugar craving – which does eventually disappear. Sweeteners have to be processed by the body, and are often broken down into less than desirable substances that can stress the immune system.

DIP INTO NATURE'S PHARMACY

Foods of plant origin obtain their characteristic colour and flavour from a rich array of compounds, known as phytochemicals. These seem to act within plants as immune system regulators by helping the plant combat dehydration, injury and viral infection. It is believed they provide similar benefits to us when we eat the plants.

Every day, the normal biochemical activity within our bodies produces dangerous molecules, known as free radicals. These free radicals can cause serious damage within cells, including genetic damage, and it is thought that they may be at least partly responsible for the changes we recognize as 'ageing'. Phytochemicals appear to combat free radicals; they also support our immune systems in overcoming infection and may, possibly, help prevent cancer.

As yet, we do not know enough about how to balance phytochemicals when taking them as supplements, and in the few experiments that have been conducted this approach has failed. However, there is very good scientific evidence of the health benefits to be gained

FIBRE-RICH FOODS

The following portions each contain about 5g (¼oz) of fibre:

- **50g (1¾oz) wholemeal flour** or uncooked pasta
- **150g (5½oz) white flour**
- **85g (3oz) raspberries**, blackberries, currants, raisins, sunflower seeds
- **75g (2½oz) cooked haricot, kidney or butter beans**, or uncooked oatmeal
- **30g (1oz) uncooked prunes**, dried figs
- **2 medium apples**, bananas, oranges or pears
- **1 corn on the cob**

when different phytochemicals are eaten as a natural mixture in a diet rich in fruit, vegetables, pulses (legumes) and whole grains. Ideally, your diet should contain 3–5 portions of vegetables and 2–4 portions of fruit each day, 1 portion being 85g (3oz).

AVOIDING A FIBRE FAMINE

Most people in Western countries eat too little fibre. Fibre has little nutritional value in its own right, as it is largely undigested, but it does promote a healthy balance of bacteria in the large bowel and makes stools more bulky. Bulky stools are passed more easily, which usually eases the symptoms of irritable bowel syndrome (IBS). Eating a diet high in fibre also reduces the risk of developing colon cancer, diverticular disease and haemorrhoids, and helps lower the level of cholesterol in the blood. You should aim for about 30g (1¼oz) of dietary fibre per day, which is easily achievable if you eat whole grains and 5–8 portions of fruit and vegetables each day.

Fat is essential to health

Dietary fat has had to take the blame for many health problems, but not all fat is the same. Different types have different chemical structures; some types are essential, which means they cannot be made in the body and have to be present in the diet, while others contribute to heart disease and should be eaten sparingly.

Ideally, intake of saturated fats, which are found in dairy products and farmed meat, should be limited. In addition, you should avoid hydrogenated fats, which are found in many types of margarine and processed foods, such as biscuits. Hydrogenated fats have been altered chemically during processing so that the body is less able to deal with them safely. Both these types of fat can aggravate inflammation and, as a result, aggravate the symptoms of eczema, asthma and arthritis.

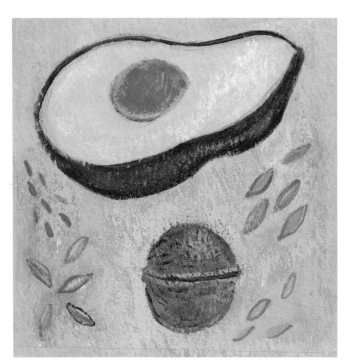

Many health-conscious people have opted to ban meat and dairy products from their diets. In many ways this is unwise, as they are valuable sources of minerals. Some fat is also essential to allow absorption of the fat-soluble vitamins, A, D and E (see p.113). You can limit

ESSENTIAL FATTY ACIDS

Omega-3 fats	Oily fish: salmon, mackerel, sardine, tuna, pilchard, anchovies. Plant sources: linseeds (flaxseeds), pumpkin seeds, walnuts, wheatgerm, rape-seeds (canola) and hemp seeds.
Omega-6 fats	Sunflower seeds, safflower seeds, sesame seeds, rapeseeds (canola), evening primrose and star flower seed oils, grape seeds, hemp seeds, soya beans and pumpkin seeds.
Omega-9 fats	Olive oil, avocado.

When extracted for supplements or cooking, unsaturated oils should be cold pressed. Keep omega-3 and omega-6 oils in dark-coloured bottles in a cool, dark place.

the amount you eat, however, by selecting small portions of lean red meat, white meat without the skin, wild game (which contains a greater proportion of unsaturated fats), fish and low-fat dairy products.

THE GOOD FATS

The essential fats are the polyunsaturated omega-3 and omega-6 fats that are needed for healthy cell membranes and to counteract inflammation, some of which can be caused by unhealthy fats. As these fats are usually liquid at room temperature, they are often called oils.

Polyunsaturated oils, however, should not be used for cooking, as they change chemically when heated or exposed to the air. This does not happen to the monounsaturated omega-9 oils, though, as they are more stable. These oils help prevent the skin becoming dry and the walls of the arteries from becoming hardened.

WHERE TO FIND HEALTHY OILS

All parts of plants contain small amounts of healthy oils – which is another reason for making sure you eat plenty of fruit and vegetables, especially green vegetables, such as spinach, purslane and kale. The highest concentrations of oil from plants, however, is found in seeds, nuts and whole grains. The omega-3 oils are also found in oily fish.

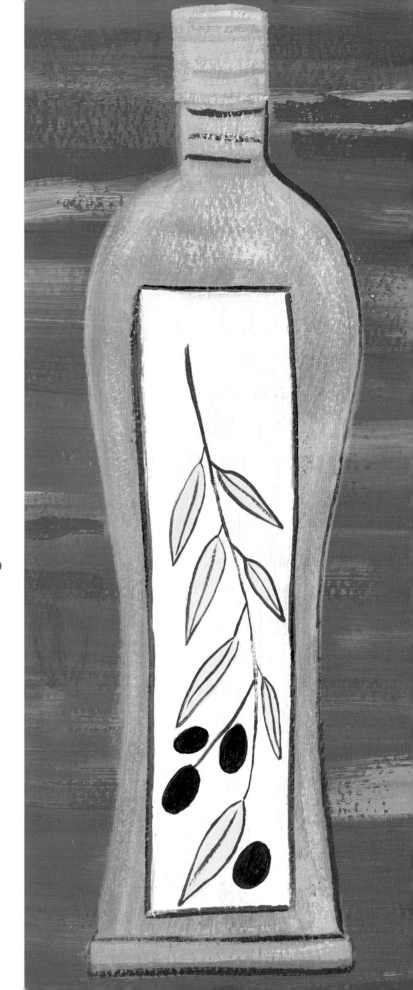

Vitamins, minerals and other supplements

There is continuing controversy about whether or not we need to take vitamin and mineral supplements. Some nutritionists believe that even the best diet may be low in essential nutrients. They believe the reason for this is that vitamins can be lost during storage or as a result of artificial ripening, and also because not all minerals are included in the chemical fertilizers used in modern farming.

If you wish to take mineral and vitamin supplements, make sure you follow these guidelines:

- **Always check the label** and never exceed the manufacturer's recommended dose. Try to avoid mixing supplements from different sources, as some vitamins and minerals are toxic. Obtain professional advice if you have to use more than one source and the total dose of an individual mineral or vitamin exceeds that given opposite.
- **While you are following the Diet Plan, choose yeast-free preparations**, and make sure that the brand you take does not contain any additives that you are excluding as part of the plan.
- **If you have a medical condition**, take regular medication, or are or might be pregnant, seek advice from your doctor or nutritionist before taking any nutritional supplements or herbal preparations.
- **Unless your nutritionist has advised otherwise, always take B vitamins** as part of a multi-vitamin preparation as the manufacturer will have balanced the doses.

PROBIOTICS AND PREBIOTICS

The normal healthy balance of micro-organisms in the digestive tract can be upset if you have food intolerance, irritable bowel syndrome or a problem with Candida. Recent research supports the theory that probiotic supplements, containing the important micro-organisms *Lactobacillus acidophilus* and *Bifidobacterium bifidum*, can reverse the imbalance. Unfortunately, these micro-organisms are delicate and do not survive well in capsules. Professor Hamilton-Miller, of the Royal Free and University College Medical School in London, recently found that only 12 out of a sample of 40 supplements contained the correct number and types of micro-organisms, as claimed on the product label. A better alternative may be to eat live yogurt that has been made with the same micro-organisms.

You can also increase the number of friendly micro-organisms in your digestive tract if you eat a fibre supplement known as fructo-oligosaccharides (FOSs). FOSs are derived from foods such as bananas, Jerusalem artichokes, onions and garlic.

SUGGESTED DOSE		BEST FOOD SOURCES
Vitamin A	2500–5000iu	Full-fat dairy products, oily fish, liver, egg yolks
Vitamin B1	5–10mg	
Vitamin B2	5–15mg	Whole grains, pulses (legumes), dried yeast, yoghurt,
Vitamin B3	10–50mg	lean meat, figs, dates, eggs, molasses, nuts, fish,
Vitamin B6	10–20mg	green leafy vegetables, apricots, pumpkins, liver,
Pantothenate	20–50mg	yeast extract
Folic acid	400–600mcg	
Vitamin B12	20–100 mcg	Liver, kidney, eggs, milk, cheese
Vitamin C	200–1000mg	Citrus fruit, kiwi fruit, green leafy vegetables, broccoli, new potatoes, sweet potatoes, bean sprouts
Vitamin D	50–400iu	Oily fish, fish liver oils, egg yolks, full-fat dairy produce
Vitamin E	60–400iu	Wheatgerm, nuts, dark green leafy vegetables, whole grains, seeds
Carotene mixture	5–20mg	Green leafy vegetables, red and orange vegetables and fruits
Calcium	300–500mg	Dairy products, nuts, seeds, broccoli, sardines, molasses
Magnesium	300–500mg	Dark green leafy vegetables, seeds, nuts, raisins, onions, molasses, mushrooms, potatoes
Iron	5–15mg	Red meat, green vegetables, seaweed, sunflower seeds (supplements are not recommended for men or post-menopausal women if they eat red meat)
Zinc	10–20mg	Nuts, seeds, meat, sardines, tuna, whole grains
Manganese	5–20mg	Nuts, green leafy vegetables, beets, egg yolks, peas
Copper	1–3mg	Liver, seafood, brewer's yeast, olives, nuts, oatmeal
Chromium	50–300mcg	Whole grains, shellfish, liver, eggs, lettuce, bananas
Selenium	50–100mcg	Wheatgerm, brazil nuts, broccoli, seafood, tomatoes
Iodine	50–100mcg	Sea vegetables, seaweed, fish, iodized salt

(NB mg=milligram, mcg=microgram, iu=international unit)

They are not digested but provide a very good food source for the micro-organisms in the digestive tract, and are known as prebiotics.

It is best to start at a low dose, as they can cause bloating, and gradually build up to the level the manufacturer recommends.

Herbal supplements

Always use any Western or Chinese herbal medicines with care and consult a therapist. Although herbal medicines can be effective, you may become allergic to the plants or ingredients used in their manufacture. Some herbs that help allergies may already be present in your diet; the rest you can obtain from health food shops.

ALOE VERA

Aloe vera enhances the immune system and reduces inflammation. It has been shown to relieve asthma, although not in people who also needed to take steroids. When applied to the skin, aloe vera aids healing, but care is needed as it can produce an allergic reaction. For advice on the correct dosage, follow the manufacturer's instructions.

VALERIAN

Valerian is used as a sedative to relieve insomnia, stress and anxiety. It can also relieve pain. Valerian is very safe, but you should not drive or operate machinery if you feel drowsy after taking it. Always follow the manufacturer's instructions as regards dosage.

MARSHMALLOW ROOT AND SLIPPERY ELM

Marshmallow root and slippery elm are soothing herbs that can be taken either together or individually to calm irritation and inflammation of the digestive tract. The dried bark of the slippery elm and/or the dried marshmallow root can be made into an infusion by being simmered in some water according to the manufacturer's instructions. Slippery elm is also sold in capsules.

MINT AND PEPPERMINT

Plants from the mint family have been used for at least 2000 years to ease digestive disturbances. Teabags are readily available, or you can infuse some fresh leaves from a home-grown plant. Peppermint oil capsules can alleviate the symptoms of irritable bowel syndrome; they have also been found to be useful in combating Candida. Inhalation of a few drops of peppermint oil diluted in hot water can relieve a runny nose in hay fever, but do not continue to use for more than a day or two without seeking professional advice.

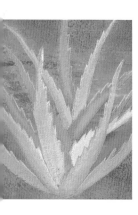

LIQUORICE

Liquorice root has long been used to calm the symptoms of asthma, eczema and rheumatoid arthritis. In addition, it can be used as a sweetener. Follow the manufacturer's instructions on dosage.

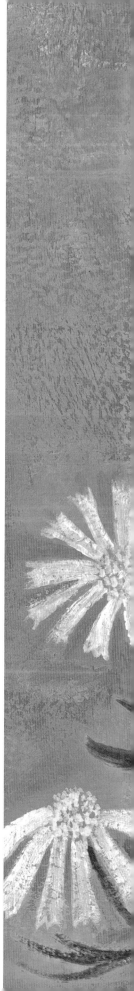

Normal culinary use of herbs is safe, but if you use a manufactured preparation make sure you:

- **Check with your doctor** first if you take any regular medication, have a medical condition, or are or might be pregnant.
- **Never exceed the dosage** recommended by the manufacturer.
- **Stop taking the herb** and seek professional advice if you notice any new symptoms.

Caution: avoid liquorice if you have a history of high blood pressure or kidney failure, as it causes fluid retention. If you wish to take liquorice for longer than 2–3 weeks, you should check with your doctor or consult a herbalist, as prolonged use can alter the balance of certain electrolytes in the blood.

TURMERIC

Turmeric, which contains curcumin, a potent antioxidant, is used in ayurvedic medicine to relieve inflamed joints in rheumatoid arthritis. Turmeric can be eaten freely in the diet, but curcumin is best taken under professional supervision, as high doses can damage the digestive tract.

THE ONION FAMILY

The phytochemicals (see p.109) that occur naturally in onions can help relieve asthma and eczema. Garlic has an anti-fungal action that can be valuable if you have a Candida problem.

FEVERFEW

Feverfew has been used for centuries to treat migraine and arthritis. Follow the manufacturer's instructions on dosage. Caution: chewing the raw leaves can cause mouth ulcers and contact with the sap can also cause an allergic reaction.

GINGER

Ginger is often used to relieve trapped wind and to counteract nausea. Steep a few slices of ginger root or ½ tsp dried ginger in boiling water, and drink as soon as it is cool enough.

FENNEL TEA OR ANISE WATER

To help dispel trapped wind in irritable bowel syndrome or food intolerance, crush 1 tsp of fennel seeds or aniseeds, place in a mug and add boiling water. Steep for 20 minutes, strain to remove the seeds and then drink the liquid.

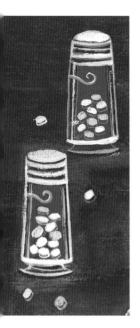

Self-help with homeopathy

Allergic symptoms often respond well to homeopathic treatment. For a cure you will usually need to consult a homeopathic practitioner (see p.146), but, if you do not have access to one, you may be able to control your symptoms yourself with homeopathic medicines bought over-the-counter.

Homeopathic medicines are made from natural substances. These substances would cause the same symptoms if you were to take them when you were well. To prevent these substances making your symptoms worse, they are diluted during their preparation as medicines. The medicines are then usually added to sugar tablets, granules or powders. The sugar used most often is lactose (from milk), but other sugars are also used and, if necessary, you can ask the pharmacist for a different sugar or for a liquid medicine.

Avoid eating, drinking, smoking or cleaning your teeth for 30 minutes before taking a homeopathic medicine and for 15 minutes afterwards. Do not touch the medicine; put the tablet (or 6–10 granules) in a spoon, and place it directly into your mouth where you should allow it to dissolve. Powders can usually be

HOME REMEDIES

What to take for hay fever, and similar allergies affecting the nose and eyes:

Allium cepa	When the discharge from the nose is profuse and burning on the upper lip. Symptoms relieved by going out of doors.
Arsenicum album	When the nose feels totally blocked, and the discharge dripping from it burns the upper lip.
Euphrasia	When the tears burn and the eyes are red, sore and itchy. The discharge from the nose is bland.
Natrum muriaticum	When you have frequent sneezing, and the discharge from the nose appears like the white of egg.
Nux vomica	When you have terrible sneezing on getting up in the morning with discharge from the nose that dries up at night.
Pulsatilla	For itchy eyes filled with tears, but relieved by cold compresses.
Sabadilla	For frequent, exhausting sneezing, with itching in the nose.
Wyethia	For intense itching of the roof of the mouth, nose and ears.

taken from the paper in which they are dispensed, but shaking them into a little water first can be helpful when giving them to a child.

If you wish to use any of the homeopathic medicines mentioned in this book use the 6c strength, and repeat the dose every 30 minutes for up to six doses, unless otherwise directed. As soon as your symptoms improve decrease the frequency of the doses and stop taking the medicine as soon as you feel better, as homeopathic medicines should not normally be used when symptoms are absent. If your symptoms seem to be getting worse stop taking the medicine – the symptoms will usually improve and may even clear completely. If your symptoms return after initially improving, you can repeat the same regime.

HOMEOPATHIC DESENSITIZATION

The potentized form of allergen to which you react can often help relieve your allergy, but always stop taking the medicine if your symptoms become worse. (Caution: you should not attempt this method if you have asthma, except under professional supervision.)

Use the 30c strength and take as follows:

House-dust mites	One dose weekly for 6 weeks, then one monthly. Stop in the summer and only restart if your symptoms recur.
Grass pollens	One dose weekly. Start 6 weeks before the season begins, and continue throughout the season (see p.27 and p.28).
Mixed moulds	As for grass pollens (see p.27 and p.28).
Tree pollens	As for grass pollens (see p.27, p.28 and p.130).

For contact allergic dermatitis:

Nickel	Take one dose every 4 weeks until symptoms subside, and repeat the course if the allergy returns.

For allergies to pets:

Cat fur **Dog fur** **Horse dander**	Take one dose weekly for 4 weeks if you come into contact with the animal frequently, and repeat the course as needed. If contact is infrequent take a dose 30 minutes beforehand, repeat every 2 hours for 4 doses, then stop. Repeat the course as needed.

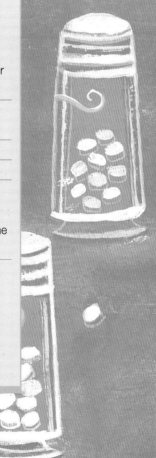

Helping yourself with exercise

Exercise provides a way of improving your mental and physical health that need not cost a penny. Physical fitness leads to a healthier heart, stronger muscles that tire less easily, increased physical flexibility, improved weight control and a slowing down of some of the physical changes of ageing. Best of all, it makes you feel better and sleep better, since a moderate, but not excessive, amount of exercise stimulates the immune system. If you are over 30, or have any health problem, it is best to check with your doctor before starting an exercise programme.

Different types of exercise have different effects and it is best to include all three of the types described here if you want to derive the greatest benefit. This does not mean that you need to undertake heroic amounts of exercise: as little as 15 minutes of physical activity twice a day on 4–5 days each week can make a big difference.

Of course, what you can do in this time depends on what sort of allergy you are combating, but if you have a regular programme, start very gently and increase your exercise gradually, you will probably be pleasantly surprised, both at what you can achieve and the improvement obtained.

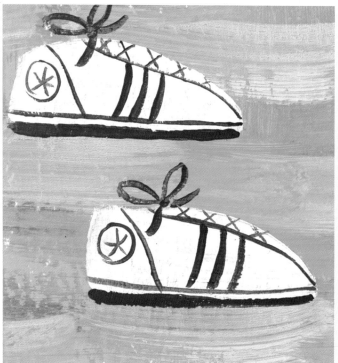

ANAEROBIC EXERCISE

Anaerobic exercise is so named because the brief periods of intense activity mean that the muscles have to use energy sources other than the oxygen in the blood. As the activity is intense, the muscles become stronger, allowing you to push, pull and lift heavy loads. In time, you also develop greater endurance so that the muscles can work for longer periods of time without tiring.

Formal examples of anaerobic exercise include weightlifting, press-ups, abdominal crunches and leg raises. Less formally, there are many anaerobic activities in daily life, such as carrying the shopping home, lifting a small child and digging the garden.

AEROBIC EXERCISE

Aerobic exercise is vigorous activity that you take for at least 12 minutes without stopping. Although you will puff a little, you should be able to continue with a conversation. If this is not possible, slow down as it is a sign that you are going too fast. A more scientific way of deciding the right level of activity for you is to take your **pulse** (see p.94). Your ideal heart rate should be about 75 per cent of its maximum rate, which can easily be calculated by subtracting your age from 220.

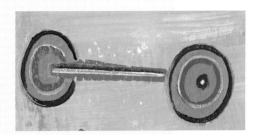

If you have a respiratory allergy you may need to wear a mask while exercising outdoors. A simple dust mask, available both at pharmacies and builder's merchants, will keep out dust and large particles, such as pollens. If you need to exclude chemicals, such as diesel and petrol fumes, you will need a more specialized mask, which can be obtained from allergy organizations. If you have asthma, a gentle stroll may be aerobic for you, but take it regularly, as you will find that you can increase both the pace and the distance. Ask your doctor for individual advice about the best times to take your medication.

If you have chronic fatigue syndrome or fibromyalgia, you will probably find that simply doing your daily chores is about as much exercise as you can manage most of the time. However, you should try to do more whenever possible because the benefits to your immune system can be great. For example, the activity of the natural killer cells in the immune system has been shown to increase by up to 100 per cent with regular exercise. **Tai chi** (see p.121) is particularly beneficial, and is likely to be aerobic if you have been doing very little exercise for some time.

Aerobic exercise includes walking briskly, jogging, aerobics classes, line or step dancing, swimming and rowing. Less formally, take the stairs instead of the lift, walk instead of using the car for short journeys and make time for a family walk every weekend.

STRETCHING

By keeping the muscle fibres long, stretching improves the ability of the joints to move fully. Muscles that extend fully are less likely to be injured or become stiff after exercise. Your posture will improve and you will probably feel better and more confident. **Yoga** (see p.120) and **tai chi** (see p.121) are both formal stretching exercises. Informally, it is often helpful to get up and stretch yourself regularly during your working day.

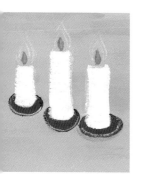

Helping yourself with yoga

Yoga was originally devised as a method of attaining spiritual development. Today, in the West, the gentle exercises and body postures of yoga are usually pursued for their physical benefits. Scientific research suggests that yoga can reduce the frequency of asthma attacks, alleviate the symptoms of rheumatoid arthritis and restore energy more effectively than visualization or relaxation (see p.124). Although there are books that describe simple yoga, it is best to join a class led by a teacher who is trained in yoga therapy. Work at your own pace and do not compete with your classmates.

BREATHING EXERCISES

The different breathing exercises practised during yoga can help with respiratory allergies such as asthma and hay fever. Many people with asthma have shallow breathing and yoga can rectify this. The 'whispering breath' exercise is one example you can try at home: sit upright in front of a lighted candle, and breathe quietly as you relax your shoulders, arms and lower jaw. Then breathe in deeply through your nose, and breathe out slowly through pursed lips. On the exhalation make the candle flame flicker gently, then breathe in again and repeat the exercise.

YOGA POSTURES

When practising yoga wear loose, comfortable clothing, have bare feet and use a non-slip mat on the floor. Never adopt postures within three hours of eating. When you are learning you will be given simple postures at first and, as you progress, you will be asked to hold the postures for longer, and stretch a little further.

THE TRIANGLE POSTURE

The triangle posture strengthens your back and stretches the muscles at the sides of your trunk:

- Stand with your feet wide apart, the right food pointing to the right and the left straight ahead. Lift your arms to the sides, level with your shoulders, keeping the palms facing down.
- Inhale, then gently exhale as you bend to the right side, sliding your right arm down the right leg and keeping your left arm pointing upwards.
- Hold the position for several breaths before returning to the original position. Repeat on the other side.

Helping yourself with tai chi

Tai chi is extremely popular in China and many Chinese begin every day with tai chi exercises. The flowing movements have been described as 'swimming on land'. Tai chi is a form of non-combative martial art, reputed to improve the flow of the chi, or life energy, through the body. It improves flexibility and has been shown by recent research to reduce stress and improve breathing. It is a particularly useful form of exercise for those with chronic fatigue syndrome.

Tai chi can be learnt at home from a video but, as the sequence of movements is important, it is better to attend a class so that an instructor can watch and correct your positions. Wear loose clothing and flat shoes, but not trainers. Lessons usually begin with a warm-up session before the tai chi movements begin. Tai chi is gentle and should not result in you becoming sore or stiff afterwards. During the movements you should be focusing on breathing properly and remaining calm and unhurried. Although your teacher may not ask if you have any illnesses, it is best to make him or her aware of your allergies. Try to practise tai chi every day; in any event you will need to incorporate it a minimum of once a week to obtain benefit from the exercises.

A SIMPLE TAI CHI EXERCISE

- Stand with your feet about shoulder width apart, knees relaxed and arms by your sides.
- Keeping your arms slightly bent and hands relaxed and facing downwards, raise your arms forward to the height of your shoulders.
- Step forward on to your right foot and bring your hands together at shoulder level, the right palm facing towards you and the left away.
- Return your arms to the same position as in the second step.
- Shift your weight back on to your left foot as you drop your hands to waist level, with palms facing down.
- Then breathe out, pushing your palms forward, at shoulder level, and move your weight on to the right foot.

121

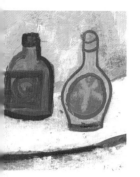

Stress management

Stress management means taking charge of all areas of your life. This requires a little effort, but if you can identify the areas where you do not cope well you are more than halfway towards learning how to cope better. In general, people are often able to manage well during a sudden crisis, but may afterwards develop symptoms of anxiety, such as palpitations, diarrhoea or sleep disturbances. These symptoms are caused by the production of the stress hormones adrenaline and cortisone, which can also adversely affect the immune system.

After a major crisis, our immune system usually recovers well, partly because other people offer help and comfort. Perversely, it is the smaller stresses of everyday life that can cause us problems. We produce small amounts of stress hormones most of the time, resulting in different symptoms (see below). At the same time, our immune system functions less effectively, with the result that, unless we take steps to manage the effects of stress, we become more prone to develop allergic symptoms.

HOW TO RECOGNIZE STRESS

You may be suffering from stress if you have three or more of the following symptoms:

- irritability, anxiety or depression.
- emotional outbursts.
- constant tiredness or disturbed sleep.
- indecisiveness or an inability to concentrate.
- inability to relax at weekends or on holiday.
- muscles that feel tense or tender, or digestive disturbance.
- frequent infections, such as coughs and colds.
- compulsive shopping.
- tendency to eat too much, drink too much alcohol, or dependency on drugs or tobacco.

HOW TO KEEP STRESS UNDER CONTROL

Making time to relax should be a priority. You should ensure that you devote 20 minutes to relaxation every day, even if you have to book it into your diary. Choose one or more ways to relax that suit you, and then make sure you take the time every day. Self-help examples include muscle relaxation and abdominal **breathing** (see p.124), **exercise** (see p.118), **meditation** (see p.124), a **leisurely bath**, scented with your favourite **aromatherapy oils** (see p.125 and p.150), or listening to your favourite music. Alternatively, treat yourself to a **massage** (see p.148) or register for a class, such as **yoga**, (see p.120) or **tai chi** (see p.121). Long walks are also helpful, especially for IBS.

Sleep is also beneficial, as it appears to be an antioxidant for the brain (see box, opposite). Try to get 6–8 hours sleep every night – we can easily recover from a few days of little sleep, but long-term sleep deprivation is thought to accelerate brain ageing and to interfere with other rejuvenation processes in the body, including the repair of the immune system.

Think about what you can do to make your work less stressful. Learn to delegate tasks, to say no to unreasonable demands and to prioritize your work. If necessary, go to some self-assertiveness classes. Try to avoid working late, as long hours can make health problems worse and you are also likely to work less efficiently. Make sure you take all your holiday entitlement and plan positive activities at weekends so that you can truly leave your work behind. Arrange to take short breaks as well as longer holidays to keep you refreshed all year round. Take time out at least once a week to go to the theatre or a concert, to visit an art gallery, or to eat out with friends.

IMPROVING YOUR SLEEP

- **Eat your last meal at least two hours before bedtime.** If you are hungry later you can snack on bananas, milk or wholemeal biscuits, as these increase the production of melatonin, a hormone that increases drowsiness.

- **Avoid stimulants** in the evening, such as caffeine, alcohol and nicotine.

- **Go to bed at a regular time**, to avoid disrupting your body clock.

- **Take regular exercise**, but not immediately before bedtime as it may increase alertness.

- **If light wakes you, use an eye mask** or heavier curtains.

- **Prepare for sleep** with a massage, a warm bath or relaxing aromatherapy oils.

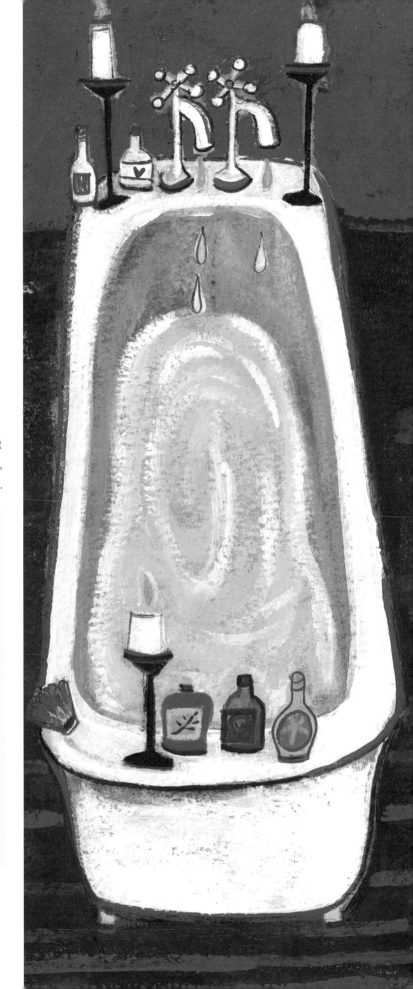

Learning to relax your muscles

When we are stressed, we hardly ever relax our muscles completely, even in our sleep. The muscles of the chest are also so tense that breathing tends to be shallow. Fortunately, we can teach ourselves to overcome these problems with abdominal breathing and muscle relaxation.

To open the lungs fully using abdominal breathing sit in a comfortable position and place one hand on your chest and the other on your abdomen. Watch the way in which each hand moves as you breathe quietly for a few minutes. Breathe in slowly through your nose and, when you finish, push out your abdomen. Notice that this enables you to take in extra air. Pause for a few seconds and then breathe out gently through your nose and empty your lungs as much as possible by pulling in your abdominal muscles. Repeat slowly several times, concentrating on keeping your muscles moving very gently, without straining.

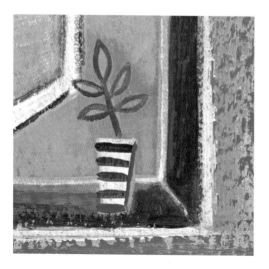

MEDITATION

Meditation reverses the effects of stress by inducing a state of relaxation and inner harmony. Although followers of most major religions practise meditation, you do not have to believe in any particular faith or philosophy to benefit from meditating. Try to incorporate meditation into your daily routine, you only need to practise for 15–20 minutes, once or twice a day to benefit from the state of calm it can bring. Check with your doctor first, however, if you have had any psychiatric problems in the past.

Although you can teach yourself to meditate by using the books, tapes and instructional videos that are now widely available, you will

VISUALIZATION

Once you have learned to relax, you can take your experience a step further with visualization, though it is best to consult a practitioner first as disturbing images can make your symptoms worse. Visualization uses the imagination to create images of your condition, the treatment you are using and the desired positive outcome.

probably find it easier if you obtain instruction from a professional. During meditation your mind requires a focus. Your focus can be a repeated phrase, sound or prayer, an object, such as a sacred or favourite picture, a vase of flowers or a lighted candle, an awareness of your breathing or even a rhythmic activity, such as tai chi or swimming.

Most people find the best way to practise meditation is adopt a comfortable position in a quiet, warm room. Breathe slowly and rhythmically, and focus your mind on your chosen phrase or object. If thoughts intrude, do not worry; try to stay as still as possible and gently bring your mind back to the focus of your meditation. End your meditation gradually, allowing yourself a few moments to become aware of your surroundings.

RELAXING WITH WATER

If one of the things you like to do is to relax in a bath after a long day, the following things can make the experience more therapeutic:

- A full-spectrum light source that replicates the light provided by the sun.
- Growing some plants that flourish in steamy bathroom conditions.
- Playing tapes that provide music or natural sounds that you find soothing, such as birdsong, wind in the trees, waves on the beach or the sound of whales.
- Redecorating in the right colour: turquoise is said to stimulate the immune system, green to treat nervous tension and blue to treat insomnia and overactivity. If in doubt consult a colour therapist.

TO RELAX YOUR MUSCLES

- Remove your shoes, loosen your clothes, lie on your back on a firm surface, with your head resting on a small pillow.
- Breathe quietly for a few minutes, pausing between each breath. If your mind wanders, do not become upset; just refocus gently on your breathing.
- Continue to breathe calmly, then tense the muscles of your right foot for a few seconds and relax them. Do the same with the muscles of the right calf, then the thigh and finally the buttock. Repeat on the left.
- Tense and release the muscles of your right arm, starting with the hand. Repeat on the left.
- Tense and release the muscles of your abdomen and then shrug your shoulders.
- Finally, tense and release the muscles of your face.
- Focus again on your breathing and relax quietly for as long as you wish.

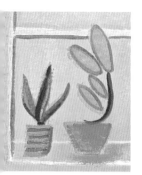

Creating a lo-allergy home and workplace

A radical increase in the amount of pollution inside buildings has led experts to consider the extent to which this may be contributing to the high levels of allergic illness, especially asthma, which has been recorded in recent years.

In our desire to minimize heating costs and improve comfort, our homes and offices have become increasingly hermetically sealed. At the same time, manufacturers have introduced many new chemicals into products such as cleaning agents, insecticides, deodorants, photocopiers, perfumes and cosmetics. Many of these are liquid and so are readily vaporized, but the process, known as 'outgassing', from those that are solid may also be significant. Outgassing is the loss, from the surface of a solid, of small numbers of molecules into the air, a process that is particularly likely to occur with modern synthetic fabrics, soft plastics and furniture glues and finishes.

The extent to which exposure to these vapours contributes to allergy is still being studied, but evidence of their ability to cause or aggravate allergy, at least in susceptible people, is steadily accumulating. There is also growing evidence that some of these chemicals are potentially irritant, toxic or even carcinogenic. Even though they may be individually safe, little is known about the effects of exposure to a cocktail of different chemicals nor has there been sufficient research into the consequences of long-term exposure.

You can reduce your exposure to these chemicals if you:

- **Ban cigarette smoke** from your home and workplace; if a special indoor area is designated for smoking in the workplace it should be ventilated with an extractor fan to the outside and smoke-polluted air should not enter the air-conditioning system.
- **Avoid air fresheners:** air your house every day by opening the windows, and at work request windows that open, especially where any chemicals are used – for example in rooms with photocopiers.
- **Minimize your use of strong-smelling chemical cleaning agents**, including fabric conditioners and aerosols. Bicarbonate of soda (baking soda) or borax dissolved in water can be used for most cleaning jobs around the home, and you can clean windows and mirrors with a solution made up of 30ml (1fl oz) vinegar to 250ml (8fl oz) water.
- **Use electric fires and cookers:** gas and paraffin appliances produce fumes.
- **Site boilers away from working or living areas**, in a separate building if possible. Position the flue to avoid fumes entering the building.
- **Seal any communicating door into an**

integral garage or to any area where chemicals, such as sprays, are used regularly.

- If you can afford to, **change an old car** if it smells of diesel or petrol. People who are chemically sensitive (see p.48) should, if possible, buy a car that is 6–12 months old, since the vapours from plastics and fabrics will have dispersed by then.

- **Hang new and recently dry-cleaned clothes outside** for a few hours before wearing or storing them in your wardrobe. Air smelly magazines and books the same way.

- **Choose solid wood furniture** or apply low toxicant sealants.

- **Avoid carpets** and fabrics that have been treated with insecticides or stain-resistant chemicals.

- **Decorate your house in the summer**, when it is possible to leave the windows open,

allowing the paint fumes to clear more quickly.

- **Reduce your use of cosmetics** as they contain dyes, preservatives and artificial fragrances.

SICK BUILDING SYNDROME

Sick (or tight) building syndrome is a relatively new phenomenon. In recent years people working in new or recently refurbished buildings have succumbed to various illnesses in greater than average numbers. As houses are built with similar materials, it is possible that the home environment could also be causing problems. Generally, people who are prone to allergies are most likely to be affected. Symptoms vary greatly, and usually include fatigue, headaches, sore throats, skin rashes and rhinitis. Improving ventilation can sometimes alleviate the symptoms.

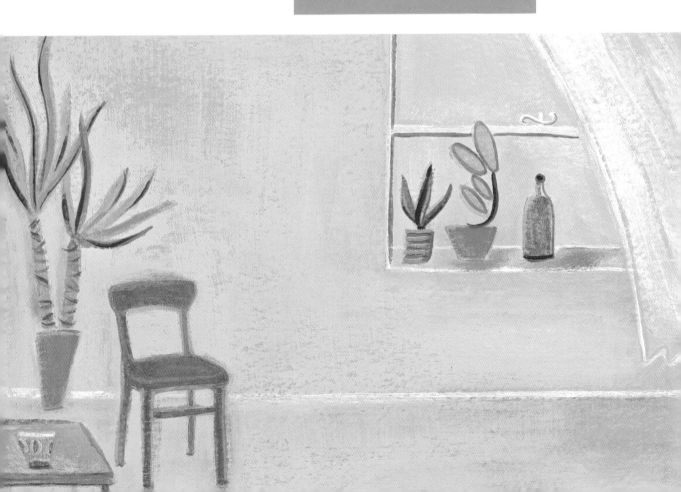

Creating a lo-allergy garden

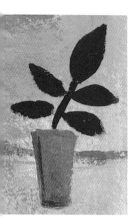

Your garden can be a dangerous place if you have allergies. Flowering plants produce pollens, other plants produce irritant sap, stinging insects make their homes there and, unless your garden is organic, you are likely to come into contact with a wide array of chemical fertilizers and pesticides.

If your symptoms are not too severe you may find that simply staying away from the culprit plants relieves your symptoms. If you choose to stay indoors during the flowering season of one or two plants remember that furry pets can bring pollen indoors. You should also inspect bunches of bought flowers carefully to ensure that you are not allergic to the pollen or sap of any of the flowers or foliage.

PLANNING THE GARDEN

Many people regard a well-maintained lawn as the centrepiece of their garden, but grass, unfortunately, is a very common source of allergens. Even if it is kept short, you will find that it can adapt by flowering very close to the ground, the flowers only being visible if you inspect the grass very carefully. In addition, some people with eczema react to the grass sap that is released during mowing, even if they are not actually doing the mowing themselves.

One alternative is to remove the lawn and replace it with either paving stones or gravel. Weeds can be suppressed by first laying a water-permeable membrane. If you choose gravel, you can create a low-maintenance garden by planting shrubs and other perennial plants through this membrane.

GENERAL MEASURES

Keep your garden tidy, and avoid wilderness areas where weeds can flourish. If your skin is sensitive, you should always wear gloves, but avoid rubber or latex as these can cause severe allergic reactions. Choose cotton-lined gloves whenever possible.

Avoid bonfires as, in addition to producing unwanted chemicals in the smoke, they can spread allergens over a large area. If you are sensitive to moulds, clear away fallen leaves and avoid having a compost heap, unless it is isolated and someone else can turn it for you. Take all your garden rubbish to the local waste site in sealed bags.

Most garden flowers are insect-rather than wind-pollinated. As a result, few of them are likely to cause you problems if you suffer from hay fever. Unless, of course, they come from the same family as plants that produce pollens to which you are allergic, in which case a **cross-reaction** may occur (see p.130). Some of the **plant families** are listed on pp.76–9, but only the edible ones, so you may need to check further in a plant guide. In general, if you have hay fever or are intolerant of edible grasses, you

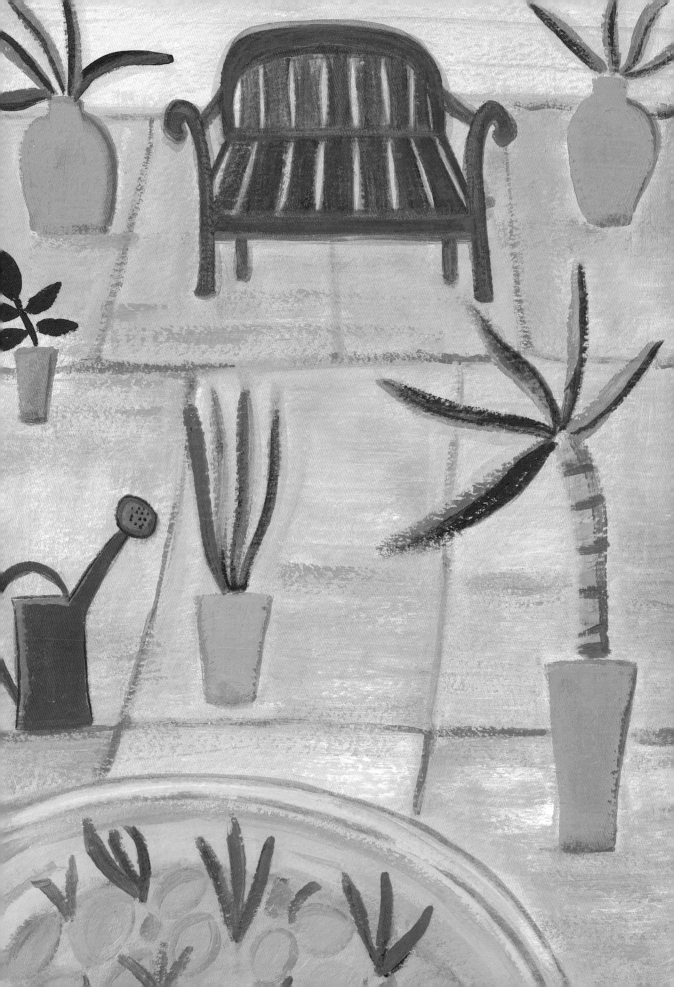

should avoid ornamental grasses. Members of the daisy family – chrysanthemums, marigolds, asters, sunflowers, goldenrod – should be avoided if you react to foods of the **daisy family** (see p.77) or are allergic to ragweed or mugwort pollens. Cross-reactions can occur, however, between plants that are unrelated (see below).

Tree pollens are more of a problem because many trees are wind pollinated. If you suffer from allergies, it is best to avoid birches, willows, alders and hazels, which produce copious pollen in late winter and early spring. Conifers are also wind pollinated and can cause hay fever symptoms when their pollen is shed.

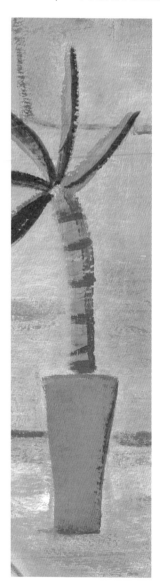

SOME CROSS-REACTIONS

If you know that you react to one of these pollens, or have had a positive allergy test to it (see p.136), you may also react to the listed food:

Pollen	Food
Birch	Apple, buckwheat, carrot, cherry, fennel, honey, peach, peanut (groundnut), pear, plum, potato, spinach, walnut, wheat
Mugwort (daisy family)	Apple, celery, carrot, melon, watermelon
Grasses	Melon, orange, Swiss chard, tomato, watermelon
Pellitory (nettle family)	Cherry, melon
Ragweed (daisy family)	Bananas, honey, melon
Pine	Pine nuts

Other cross-reactions:

Allergen	Food
House-dust mite	Kiwi fruit, papaya
Rubber	Some fruits, including bananas and cherries
Crustaceans and molluscs	This is rare and may be due either to foods that they both eat or to preservatives added by food manufacturers

Helping your baby

If there is a tendency towards allergies in your family you may be able to reduce the risk of your child developing allergic symptoms by taking some precautions. A number of factors, including low birth weight, can increase the risk of a baby developing asthma and other allergies. Measures that you can take are listed below.

- **Ideally, both parents should prepare for pregnancy by stopping smoking** and eating as healthy a diet as possible at least three months before stopping contraception, as it takes at least 100 days for sperm to develop, during which time good nutrition is vital.
- **During the pregnancy, the mother should eat as varied a diet as possible**. Some of the foods most likely to cause allergy (see box) may cross the placenta, but there is little scientific evidence to support this. If you plan to exclude all of them from your diet, you should seek professional advice from a dietitian to ensure that you obtain adequate nutrients; you should also ask about taking a calcium supplement.
- **Do not expose the baby to tobacco smoke** for at least a year, as it seems to 'turn on' the tendency to develop allergies.
- **Breastfeed for a year**, if possible, as breast milk contains antibodies that provide protection against infection. For some reason that is not understood, a baby can, on rare occasions, become allergic to its mother's milk. It is normal, however, for breastfed babies to grow more slowly than bottle-fed babies, so if your reason for giving up breastfeeding is slow growth, seek professional advice first. Breastfeeding mothers should avoid the foods

FOODS TO AVOID

Foods likely to cause allergic reactions are: milk, eggs, peanuts (groundnuts), fish, citrus fruits, wheat, beef, chicken and any food to which a previous child has been allergic.

listed in the box. Your doctor may recommend that you take a calcium supplement and obtain advice from a dietitian. If you find this approach too restrictive, remember it is better to eat normally than give up breastfeeding.

- **Do not introduce mixed feeding until the baby is 4–6 months**, as its digestive system is immature and may allow the absorption of incompletely digested proteins. These can act as allergens. For at least nine months, avoid giving the baby the foods listed in the box. Introduce new foods one at a time so that any reaction can be noted and, if necessary, the food withdrawn for a while. Avoid giving new foods when the child is ill, as infections or diarrhoea increase the likelihood that the baby will become sensitive to the food.
- **In the first year avoid exposure to environmental allergens**, such as **pollen and moulds** (see p.27), **dust-mites** (see p.19) and **furry animals** (see p.14). Avoid unnecessary surgery.

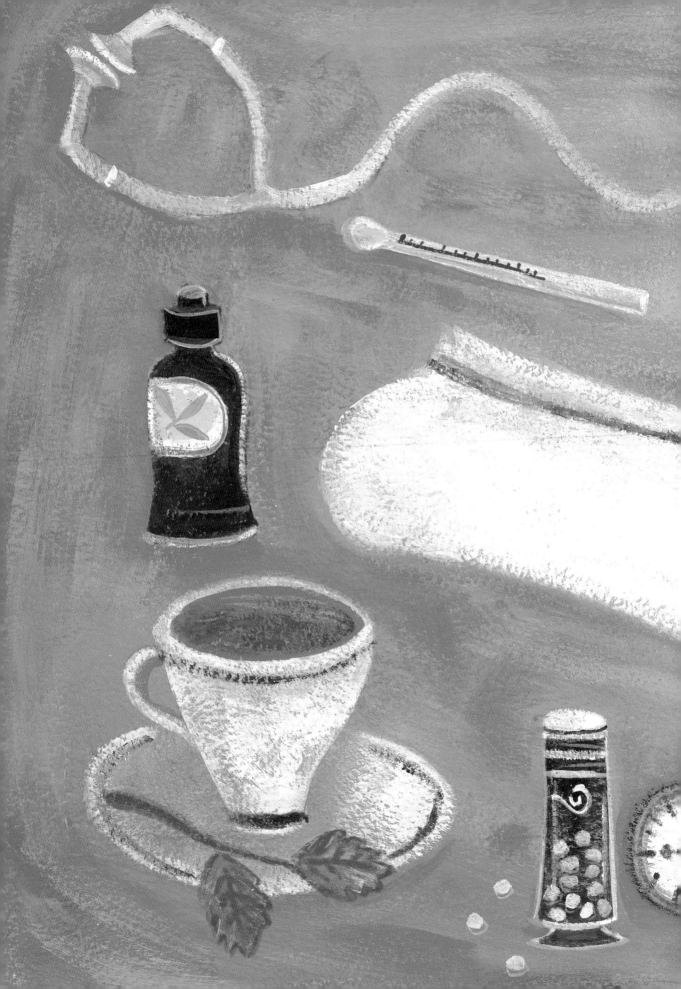

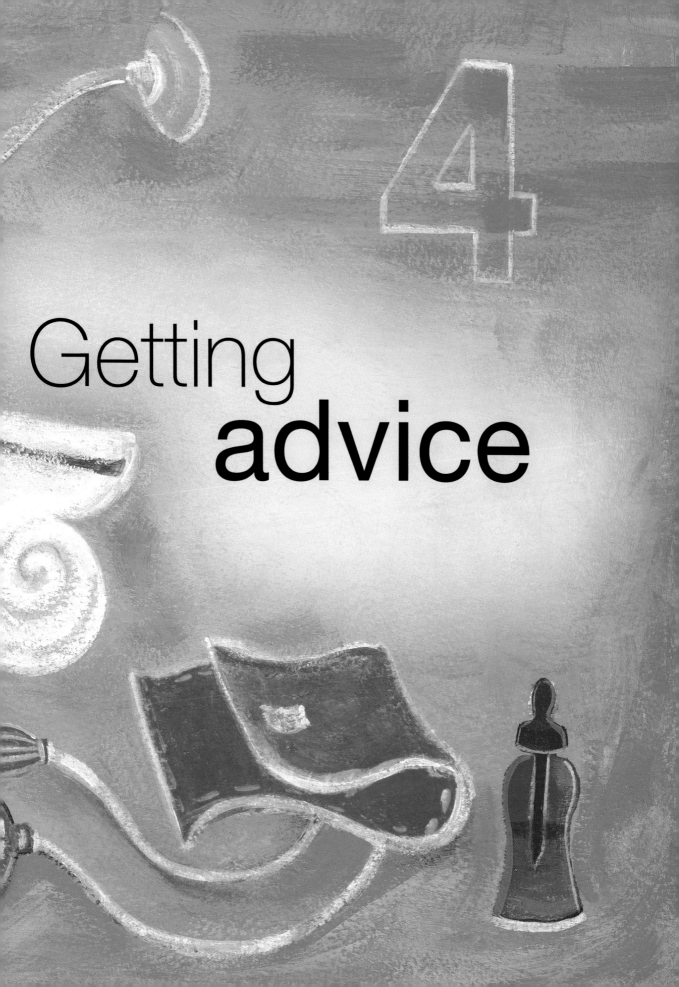

4

Getting advice

Integrated medicine

Integrated medicine reflects the growing recognition of the benefits to be had of combining Western medical and surgical techniques with complementary or alternative therapies. Where such an approach is followed, doctors, therapists and patients work together to restore health – of the mind and spirit as well as the body. Mounting evidence suggests that sufferers of allergies can benefit enormously.

CONVENTIONAL ALLERGISTS

Our knowledge of the immune system and the way it works has increased greatly in recent years. The immune system consists of various specialized cells and proteins, known as antibodies, which can recognize and respond to any incoming allergens. During this response, various chemical substances, such as histamine, are released, causing inflammation and attracting a number of different immune system cells and chemicals to reinforce the body's defences.

Immunologists have identified four basic types of allergic response, each of which has a different mechanism. It is these responses that cause the symptoms that we recognize as allergies, and conventional allergists are doctors who believe that it is incorrect to classify symptoms as 'allergic' unless these mechanisms are involved in their production. They use a number of tests (see p.136) to confirm the diagnosis and often the allergen. They advise that the allergen should, where possible, be avoided and prescribe drugs to suppress the symptoms.

ENVIRONMENTAL ALLERGISTS

Environmental allergists, who are also known as clinical ecologists, are doctors who start by trying to establish what environmental influences are the cause of the patient's symptoms, by observing whether the symptoms improve or disappear when exposure to the environmental trigger ceases. They believe that people respond to environmental triggers in one of two ways. 'Type A' allergy covers broadly the same group of illnesses that are termed 'allergies' by conventional allergists. The other response is usually called 'intolerance' or, sometimes, 'Type B' allergy. The latter is not, at present, thought to involve the immune system.

This conventional distinction between allergy and intolerance has been observed throughout this book, even though some environmental allergists suspect that in intolerance the immune system may be involved in some way that has not been established. Confusingly, most complementary practitioners refer to 'allergy' when in fact the condition they are describing is intolerance. This can cause problems for their patients, who find that doctors are dismissive because they do not accept that the condition is an allergy.

A major problem for environmental allergists is the lack of skin and blood tests for confirming the diagnosis of intolerance. As a result, making a firm

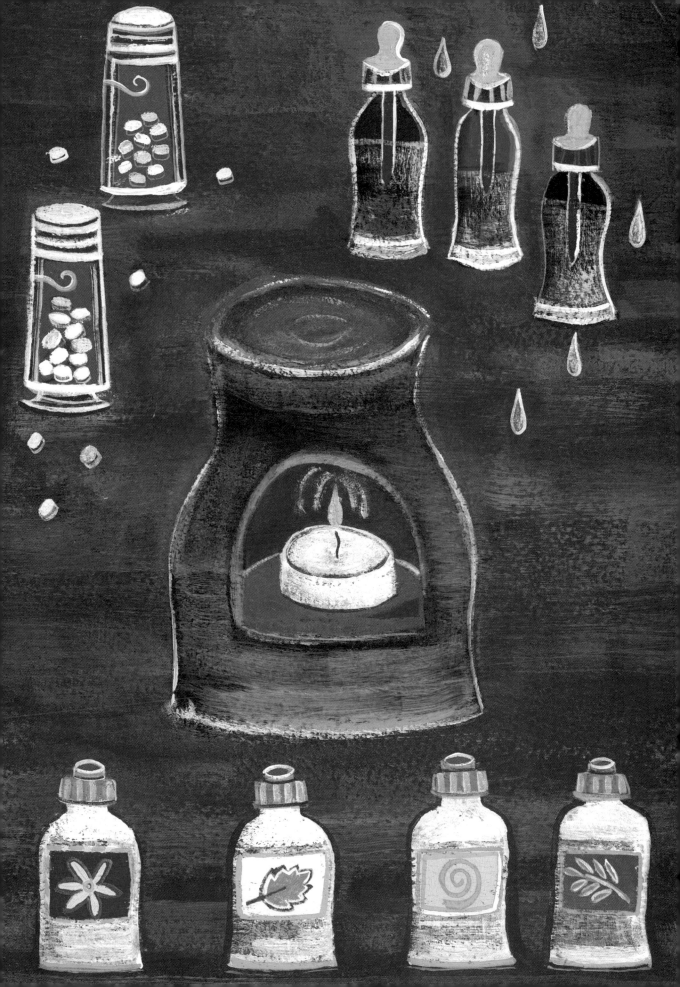

and scientifically acceptable diagnosis is almost impossible, as it depends on patients being able to recognize some sort of pattern in the development of their symptoms. This can be less easy than it sounds, as the symptoms often occur some time after exposure to the trigger, or when some sort of tolerance level has been exceeded. In addition, more than one trigger can be involved.

Environmental allergists treat intolerance by excluding the triggers. It is possible to reintroduce the triggers without causing the symptoms to return, but this may take months. The lack of symptoms is sometimes known as tolerance and can be maintained indefinitely provided exposure to the trigger is infrequent. Environmental allergists have also developed a number of other methods of treatment (see opposite page) for both Type A allergies and intolerance.

FOOD CRAVINGS

One very odd aspect of food intolerance, which does not occur with food allergy, is the fact that about 50 per cent of people with food intolerance crave the culprit food(s). Exclusion of the food(s) causes withdrawal symptoms, as in any true addiction, and reintroduction of the food at a later date can trigger the cravings again if the food is eaten too frequently. The reason for this craving is not fully understood, but it may be caused by the formation of morphine-like chemicals during the digestion of the culprit food(s). Whatever the cause, continuing to eat the food(s) is stressful to the body and appears to use up energy. Exclusion of the culprit food(s) allows energy levels to improve and other symptoms, such as poor concentration and abdominal bloating, to disappear.

Testing for allergies

The substances that cause an allergy are sometimes obvious. For example, the symptoms of hay fever occur when grasses are in flower and disappear at the end of the season. More often, tests need to be performed to find out the exact cause of the symptoms, but allergy testing is, at best, only 70–80 per cent reliable.

The first line of investigation is often skin testing, of which there are three main types:
• **Prick testing**, where a small amount of an allergen is injected into the top layer of the skin.
• **Intradermal (intracutaneous) testing**, in which slightly more allergen is injected a little deeper. This is more accurate, but can occasionally provoke a severe reaction.
• **Patch testing** for contact allergens (see p.25).

The first and second tests are positive when a red flare and small raised weal occur within about 10 minutes. They are fairly reliable for certain types of allergen, especially those that are inhaled, but are poor at detecting food allergies and intolerance, and can register positive in people who do not have any allergic symptoms. They can also give a negative result when there is a genuine allergy.

ALLERGY PREVENTION AND CURE

Desensitization: For many years, the usual treatment to prevent allergic reactions to a known allergen, such as grass pollen, was a course of injections of very tiny amounts of the allergen. The dosage was increased very slowly, until the patient could tolerate the level of allergen present in the environment. Although it was effective, severe and sometimes fatal reactions occurred. In the United Kingdom, this treatment is now only used to desensitize patients who have had serious reactions to a single allergen, such as a **bee sting** (see p.14), and it is always given in a hospital where resuscitation equipment is available.

Neutralization: Many environmental allergists now use this method. Very low dosages of the allergen or substance causing intolerance are self-administered, by injection or under the tongue, to induce **tolerance** (see p.136). To establish the dosage, the doctor injects a range until the one that does not produce a reaction is found. Treatment is continued for several months or even years, until tolerance is achieved. This method is in regular use by over 2000 doctors in the United States and only a few mild reactions have been reported.

Enzyme potentiated desensitization (EPD) is an effective treatment for a wide range of allergies, and has been in use for 30 years with few side effects being reported. A single low dosage of the allergen is 'potentiated' by being mixed with the enzyme beta glucuronidase. This dose is either injected or, for very sensitive patients, placed on to an area of skin that has previously been scraped with a blunted scalpel. The treatment is repeated every 2–3 months until the allergy subsides.

OTHER TESTS

The **pulse test** (see p.98) has been used since the 1940s. It appears to be fairly reliable, although conventional allergists would disagree. Many practitioners and some doctors use applied kinesiology, in which the patient either holds a glass phial containing the substance being tested or a little is placed under the tongue. The strength of the patient's muscles is then tested. If they weaken, the patient is said to be intolerant of the substance. This test appears to produce good results with some people. Acupuncturists claim that the electrical resistance of the skin alters after contact with an allergen or substance causing intolerance. Various methods, such as the Vegatest, have been developed to measure these changes, but their reliability is questionable.

BLOOD TESTS

The RAST (radioallergosorbent) test, which measures the amount of certain antibodies in the blood, is reliable, but does not distinguish between allergy and contact with substances that act to release **histamine** (see p.73), so is not useful for intolerance. Other blood tests that appear to provide helpful results for intolerance and allergy have been developed, but they are not consistently reliable.

Taking it further

Fifty years ago virtually all complementary and alternative therapies were dismissed by doctors, and by the majority of the population, as being useless or even dangerous. Today, most people, and even some doctors, admit to being interested in some form of non-orthodox medicine and practitioners can be found in most towns.

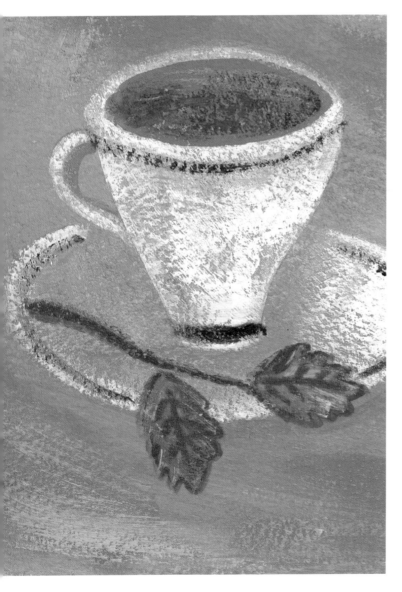

Many people turn to complementary medicine because they believe that practitioners of alternative therapies give them more time and take a greater interest in the whole person than conventional doctors. As part of this holistic approach therapists tend to ask more 'why' questions than doctors usually do. For example, in taking a history, they are often seeking to answer the question, 'Why has this disease or disorder occurred in this person at this time?' By contrast, doctors often place greater emphasis on reaching a diagnosis, and appear to concentrate more on identifying the symptoms, and when and where they occur. Conventional doctors have long accepted, however, that illness can have psychological and emotional origins, although in the past, when planning the treatment, they have often regarded these as incidental.

CONNECTING THE MIND AND THE BODY

In the past 20 years or so psychologists, doctors and other scientists have gained greater understanding of the complex relationship between the emotional and the physical aspects of people. For example, it has been shown that white cells, which

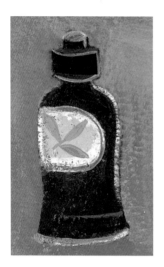

normally act to kill viruses, are less able to perform this important task in a person who is grieving. This increases the risk of that person developing a viral illness, and so provides a possible scientific explanation for the observation that people can appear to die from a 'broken heart'. Research such as this has led a growing number of conventional health practitioners to seek ways in which their patients can benefit from more than one type of therapy, and to recognize the value of an integrated approach.

This approach is still in its infancy, however. Doctors are still cautious about referring their patients, as their knowledge of alternative therapies is often limited, and the training of therapists is not always standardized. Any therapy that is powerful enough to heal is also powerful enough to harm, and just because a therapy is 'natural' does not mean that it is safe when used incorrectly.

CHOOSING A THERAPY AND A THERAPIST

- **Before starting non-conventional treatment, always consult your doctor**, so that you can discuss the best way to approach your problem. If you are pregnant or trying to conceive, it is essential to discuss any proposed alternative treatment with your doctor beforehand.
- **Choose a therapist who is fully trained and registered** with an appropriate professional organization. If possible, talk to the therapist before making an appointment to determine whether the therapy will be beneficial for your condition, how many appointments are likely to be needed, and whether or not they carry indemnity insurance.
- **If possible, talk to people who have previously consulted the same therapist**, as this will help you to assess whether they are someone with whom you will feel comfortable. Be wary of any therapist who insists that you stop conventional treatment, or asks you to change any belief system or religion.
- **Do not stop or alter the dosage** of any prescribed medication without first consulting your doctor. When appropriate, keep your doctor informed about any medication or treatment recommended by your therapist, and tell your therapist about any prescribed medication that you are taking.
- **Tell your therapist if you develop new symptoms** after starting treatment, and consult your doctor if the symptoms persist.
- **Certain types of alternative treatment are unsuitable for babies** and small children. Ask your doctor for advice if you have any doubts about proposed therapies for them.

Which therapy?

Complementary and alternative therapies can be used for the relief of symptoms but also to restore inner harmony so that your body can start to heal. This dual approach is of particular importance in the treatment of allergies, as it is almost impossible to escape completely from the allergens that cause the symptoms, so strengthening the natural defences of the body becomes essential.

A number of different therapies are described here. Some are traditional therapeutic systems that have evolved over thousands of years. These use the everyday tools that were available to the practitioners who developed them, such as herbs, massage, various methods of bodily cleansing, dietary changes and counselling. Other therapies are more modern, but in many cases they have borrowed or refined traditional methods of healing.

Chinese herbalism

Chinese herbalism is part of traditional Chinese medicine, which adopts a holistic approach to healing including exercise, such as **tai chi** (see p.121) and **acupuncture** (see p.143). Traditional Chinese medicine seeks to restore and maintain harmony and balance within the body, by choosing the most appropriate mix of therapies.

Chinese herbalism has shown to be particularly successful in alleviating eczema. The herbs are usually prescribed as a formula containing 10–15 different herbs. These are chosen after a consultation that lasts up to an hour, during which the doctor takes your medical history and gives you a physical examination that differs from the conventional Western approach in its particular interest in the pulse and the appearance of the tongue. Although Chinese herbs have been in use for many centuries modern analysis has revealed that some of them may not be totally safe, and one or two have been banned in some Western countries.

CAUTIONS

Always consult a practitioner who is fully qualified to prescribe Chinese herbal medicine. If you are pregnant, or have a history of liver disease, including hepatitis, always check with your doctor first. If you notice any new symptoms or your allergic symptoms worsen, obtain advice promptly. See also **Choosing a therapist**, p.139.

Alexander technique

The Alexander technique was developed by an Australian actor, F. M. Alexander, as a way of overcoming the stresses and strains imposed on his voice and body through acting. It eases allergic conditions by aiding stress management and restoring balance within the body.

The Alexander technique, which is suitable for all ages, is usually taught on a one-to-one basis. Your teacher will start by assessing your posture and way you normally move about. You will then be taught how to correct your posture and move in ways that do not strain your muscles.

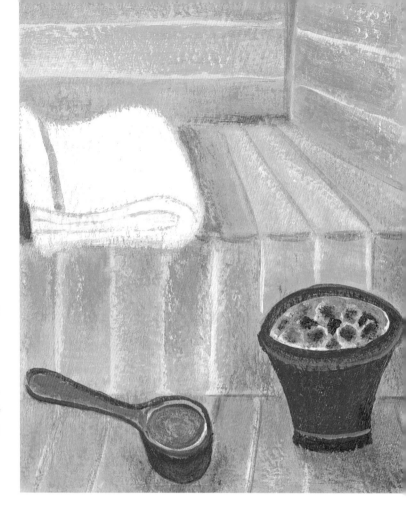

Ayurveda

Ayurveda is a traditional holistic medical system from the Indian subcontinent. Practitioners believe that illnesses, including allergies, result from an imbalance in the natural energy of the body, and that health will return when the balance has been restored. After a consultation that may last an hour or more, ayurvedic treatment usually begins with a purification regime that includes enemas, laxatives, therapeutic vomiting, saunas and massage with oils. This is then followed by a programme designed to restore health, which may include herbal remedies, yoga, chanting, meditation and sitting in the sun.

CAUTIONS

Make sure your practitioner is fully qualified to treat you with herbs. If you are pregnant, check with your doctor first. If you notice any new symptoms or your allergic symptoms worsen, obtain advice promptly. Enemas and purgatives should be avoided if you are pregnant, elderly or have heart disease; they should not be applied to infants either. See also **Choosing a therapist**, p.139.

Autogenic training

Autogenic training consists of six mental exercises that calm the mind and offer a method by which you can relax at will, and help your body to heal itself and overcome allergies. It is taught in eight weekly sessions, either on a one-to-one basis, or in small groups of 6–8 people. It can be particularly helpful in relieving stress, IBS and asthma. The practitioner will ask about your medical and psychological history, before teaching you the mental exercises that induce complete relaxation. You will need to practise the technique between classes, for about 15 minutes, three times a day.

CAUTIONS

If you have had psychological problems in the past, check with your doctor first. Tell the practitioner if you are pregnant, have a heart condition or diabetes. See also **Choosing a therapist**, p.139.

Healing and touch

Healers believe they are able to activate the natural healing mechanisms that we all have within our bodies, by directing healing energy towards the patient by means of thought or prayer, either through the laying on of hands or through distance healing. Although there is no scientific explanation for it, this type of healing has been used in many different cultures, often as part of religious practice.

Although it could be the result of the patient's own belief that healing will occur, scientific research has shown that benefits can follow the intervention of a healer. Some studies have shown changes in patients' brainwave patterns during healing. At the very least, healing offers comfort for people for whom other forms of treatment have little or nothing to offer and this relief from anxiety may itself benefit the immune system. Chronic pain and

stress-related conditions, including headaches and migraines, are the areas in which healing appears to be the most helpful.

If you consult a practitioner, you will be asked a number of informal questions about your condition. Ideally, you should feel comfortable with the healer and his/her philosophy. Healers often use their hands for healing, and may work alone or with the support of other people as, for example, during a Christian service. Patients report sensations of warmth, cold, tingling or dizziness.

CAUTIONS

Avoid healers who charge excessive amounts, promise a cure or who suggest that healing has failed to take place because of your lack of faith. See also **Choosing a therapist**, p.139.

THERAPEUTIC TOUCH

Practitioners of therapeutic touch (TT), which is a modern healing technique, believe that the body has unique energy fields that become disrupted by illness. By using their hands to touch their patients, they believe they can restore balance and enable natural self-healing to occur. TT is widely practised by nurses in the United States and is becoming popular in Britain and Australia.

CAUTIONS

Special care is needed in treating babies, also those who are pregnant, elderly or emaciated, have suffered a serious psychological illness, such as psychosis, or had a head injury or other shock. See also **Choosing a therapist**, p.139.

Biofeedback

The ability to alter the action of the autonomic nervous system, which controls blood pressure and the smooth muscles in the intestine and blood vessels, has been practised by yogis for many centuries (see also **chiropractic**, p.145).

In the 1960s, United States scientists began to use instruments that could detect changes in the autonomic nervous system through readings on a dial or a series of electronic flashes or bleeps. The scientists discovered that people could learn how to alter these readings when they were attached to the instruments, and the technique became known as biofeedback.

Biofeedback has been used to treat a number of conditions, including stress, migraines, IBS and asthma. Today, sophisticated computer programmes allow patients to control images on a VDU by altering the function of their autonomic nervous systems. The equipment is expensive, however, and you will need a practitioner to teach you the technique.

CAUTIONS

Always consult your doctor before altering the dosage of any medication that you are taking See also **Choosing a therapist**, p.139.

Acupuncture

Acupuncture is part of traditional Chinese medicine. The practitioner inserts very fine needles into specific points on the body to relieve a range of disorders, including asthma, hay fever, muscular pain and migraines. It can also be used instead of anaesthetic during surgery.

The stimulation of acupoints is believed to activate the flow of energy through the body, and restore the balance that is lost in ill health. On your first visit, you will be asked questions about your general condition and lifestyle as part of the traditional Chinese approach to assessment, which also includes a detailed physical examination. After this the needles are inserted to different depths and for varying amounts of time. They may be twisted gently to increase their effect.

Other acupuncture techniques include cupping, whereby a vacuum is created in a glass cup which is then placed on your skin over an acupuncture point, and moxibustion, which is the application of heat to one or more acupoints.

CAUTIONS

Ensure that your practitioner is fully qualified, and that she or he either sterilizes the needles in an autoclave or uses disposable ones. Always tell them if you are pregnant, or if there is a possibility you might be, and whether you have a sexually transmitted disease, such as hepatitis or AIDS. Eating, drinking alcohol, having a hot bath or shower and strenuous exercise, either immediately before or after treatment, may counteract its effect. See also **Choosing a therapist**, p.139.

ACUPRESSURE

Acupressure is the application of pressure, using the thumb or finger, to the acupuncture points, in order to stimulate healing. Ideally, you should consult a practitioner, who will take account of your medical history. Acupressure can, however, be self-administered, to relieve nausea, migraine, fatigue and digestive disorders, including IBS.

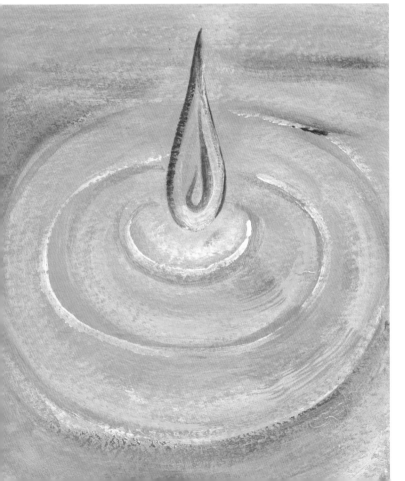

CAUTIONS

There are certain acupressure points that should be avoided during pregnancy. See also **Choosing a therapist**, p.139.

Naturopathy

Although naturopathy or 'natural medicine' was only formally developed in the late 19th century, it incorporates healing techniques that are far older. Today, conventional doctors have adopted many of its principles and methods. Naturopaths believe that the body's natural state is one of health, that the body is its own best healer and that it will always strive to achieve health. The body's underlying equilibrium can be disturbed, naturopaths believe, by a build-up of 'toxins' – waste products that can accumulate as the result of an unhealthy lifestyle and compromise the efficiency of the immune system. Many of the approaches they adopt to combat the factors that contribute to loss of health are described elsewhere in this book. These include eating a **healthy diet** (see pp.106–13), obtaining sufficient **sleep** (see p.123), taking regular **exercise** (see p.118), making sure that you get plenty of fresh air, and **reducing your exposure to pollutants** (see p.48 and p.126) and emotional or physical **stress** (see p.122).

Naturopaths adopt a multi-disciplinary approach that involves improving digestion and circulation, enhancing the elimination of waste products and boosting the immune system. Treatments are designed to be as non-invasive as possible and may include dietary changes, **yoga** (see p.120), as well as a number of therapies individually described in this section, such as **herbalism** (see p.140 and p.153) or **homeopathic medication** (see p.146), **massage** (p.148) and **hydrotherapy** (p.147).

The first consultation with a naturopath takes about an hour, and usually includes a physical examination. As a result of this, the practitioner may suggest you undergo some investigations, which can include tests used by conventional doctors, such as X-rays, as well as less conventional ones, such as analysis of hair and sweat. The treatment programme will be tailored to your individual needs and very often will involve cleansing or detoxification, via fasting, or measures to increase the discharge of waste products through sweating. It is also likely to involve treatment to reverse any perceived weakness, through an improved diet and nutritional supplements.

CAUTIONS
Avoid fasting or extreme dietary restriction unless your naturopath is fully qualified to supervise you. See also **Choosing a therapist**, p.139.

Manipulative therapies
For more than a century, chiropractors have used manipulative treatment to maintain and restore the health of the central nervous system, which serves all the organs of the body. In particular, chiropractic can affect the way the autonomic nervous system works. This system controls the action of the tiny muscles in the walls of the blood vessels, which are involved in the development of **migraine** (see p.40), the air passages, which are narrowed in **asthma** (see p.30), and the digestive system, which can be disordered in **IBS** (see p.34). (See also **autogenic training**, p.141.)

During your first consultation, which generally lasts about an hour, your chiropractor will take a detailed medical history and will ask questions about your lifestyle. He or she will also give you a physical examination, which may include taking your blood pressure and X-rays. If test results are needed first, treatment may not start until a second, shorter consultation. The practitioner will then use precise and well-controlled techniques to adjust your spine and pelvis.

Osteopaths use a variety of techniques of touch and manipulation to enhance wellbeing and reduce pain. The osteopath concentrates more on treating the soft tissues, such as the muscles, for the restoration of health and full mobility, than on joints. Although osteopathic consultations are most frequently sought for the reduction of pain, their methods can also improve allergic conditions such as migraines, asthma and digestive disorders.

Osteopathic consultations are similar in length and style to those with a chiropractor. Treatment consists of gentle manipulations and various types of massage. Your osteopath may also recommend certain relaxation techniques and exercises for you to practise between consultations.

CAUTIONS

Tell your practitioner if you have any bone conditions, such as osteoporosis, tumours or previous fractures, or any inflammation, infection or circulatory problems, such as an aneurysm. See also **Choosing a therapist**, p.139.

Homeopathy

Homeopathic medicines are made from natural substances that, if you took them when you were well, would result in the same symptoms as those caused by your illness. This basic principle of healing has long been recognized by non-Western healing traditions, including those of Indian and Mayan cultures. It also finds a mention in the teaching of Hippocrates. In many conditions, especially allergies, the symptoms can be regarded as the result of the body's attempt to heal itself. By slightly increasing the symptoms, homeopathy appears to enable the body to heal itself more effectively. To prevent your symptoms becoming worse as a result of the treatment, homeopathic medicines are very dilute. Most conventional doctors are sceptical of homeopathy, as the dosages are so small, and the medicines are often diluted to a point at which none of the original substance is left. Homeopaths, however, believe that the

method by which the medicines are made leaves an electromagnetic pattern on the diluted liquid, which is able in some way to interact with the body.

A homeopathic practitioner will take a full medical history in order to find a medicine that suits not only your symptoms but also your physical build and mental and emotional characteristics. This is called the constitutional medicine, which homeopaths believe can cure a number of allergic conditions. Many people, however, become skilled in treating their own allergies with 'local' medicines (see p.116).

CAUTIONS

Some homeopaths are also doctors, but if you are consulting one who is not medically qualified always check with your doctor if you have any unexplained symptoms, in case further conventional investigations are needed.

Ask for lactose-free medicines if you are allergic to milk. Occasionally, symptoms can become worse after treatment – something that can be a particular problem in the treatment of eczema. If this situation persists, ask your practitioner or doctor for advice. See also **Choosing a therapist**, p.139.

ANTHROPOSOPHICAL MEDICINE

Rudolf Steiner was a homeopathic doctor who founded anthroposophical medicine in the early 1900s. He believed that the natural world is guided by cosmic rhythms and that each individual has a unique purpose, a belief that was at odds with the scientific view of the day that the body was a purely physical entity. He developed a holistic approach to the treatment of a range of illnesses, including allergies. He included movement and artistic therapies, such as painting and sculpture, massage and hydrotherapy, as well as the use of anthroposophical medicines, which are made from plant, animal and mineral substances. The plants are grown and harvested in accordance with a system of 'biodynamic' agriculture that takes into account the influence of the sun, moon and other cosmic factors. All practitioners are qualified doctors.

FLOWER REMEDIES

Dr Edward Bach (pronounced batch) was an English doctor who believed that negative emotions could give rise to physical illness. He also believed that plants had healing properties which could be used to remedy various ailments. More recently, the inclusion of a wider variety of plants from around the world has increased the range of available remedies. The effects of the flower remedies are very subtle, but the action is believed to be closer to homeopathy than herbalism. Many practitioners, and also now some doctors, prescribe flower remedies at times of crisis or to treat moods such as fear and anger. It is this relief from stress that may enable the body to overcome allergic conditions.

BIOCHEMIC TISSUE SALTS

Dr Wilhelm Schüssler, a homeopathic doctor, was one of the first to suggest that illness can result from mineral deficiencies. He believed that taking the potentized form of the mineral could reverse the deficiency. He chose 12 homeopathic medicines derived from mineral sources, including rock salts and quartz, and recommended their use in low-potency dosages in which some, but only very little, of the original mineral remained. Although there is no evidence to suggest that such low dosages of 'tissue salts' are sufficient to replace a dietary deficiency, it is possible that they may influence the way in which the normal dietary supply of these minerals is absorbed and used by the body. In addition, their method of preparation means that they have an independent action as homeopathic medicines. They are widely available for self-medication as localized remedies to relieve various allergic conditions, including hay fever, asthma, and irritable bowel syndrome.

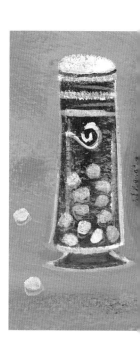

Hydrotherapy

In hydrotherapy, water is used, externally and internally, in all its forms – hot, cold and as liquid, steam or ice – to restore and maintain health. The cleansing potential of water has been recognized for many centuries and in many different medical traditions. Today, hydrotherapy is usually practised at spas and health farms. In addition to drinking spa water, which is

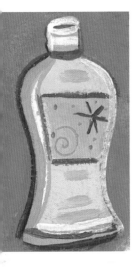

often rich in minerals, you may have a number of treatments prescribed including:

- **High-powered jets of hot or cold water** directed at your back for 2–3 minutes. Taking cold showers on a regular basis appears to enhance the action of the immune system, since the people who do so are less prone to develop respiratory infections in winter.
- **Baths of different temperatures**, including sitz baths, in which heat can be applied to one part of your body at the same time that cold is applied elsewhere. Various substances may be placed in the water to enhance the therapeutic effect of bathing. These include herbs and aromatherapy oils, which can ease respiratory allergies, Epsom salts, to enhance sweating (see below) or reduce inflammation around a joint, oatmeal to soothe the skin in eczema or urticaria, and various mineral muds and extracts, such as peat or Dead Sea salts.
- **Saunas, steam rooms and cabinets**, and Turkish baths. These may be prescribed to enhance the expulsion of waste products through increased sweat (see naturopathy).
- **Sea water and seaweed treatments** to enhance cleansing and promote relaxation.
- **The application of hot and cold wraps** and compresses. These improve circulation, stimulate the immune system, and can relieve long-term fatigue.

CAUTIONS

Avoid hot baths or steam if you have heart disease or high blood pressure. Avoid steam treatment or sitz baths during the first three months of pregnancy. In later pregnancy, limit steam treatment to 10 minutes. Avoid steam treatment just after an operation, and if you have asthma, epilepsy or a history of thrombosis. Avoid contact with seaweed if you are allergic to iodine. Do not add ingredients to a bath if you have an open wound, except under professional guidance. See also **Choosing a therapist**, p.139.

Massage

Massage releases physical and emotional tension, slows the heart rate, lowers blood pressure and relaxes the muscles. It can help release the body's natural painkillers – endorphins, and reduce levels of the stress hormones that can weaken the immune system, and which may be one reason for the development of allergic conditions. Today, there is a baffling array of different types of massage to choose from, which offer varying benefits. Massage is also being incorporated with increasing frequency into conventional treatment programmes.

Western or Swedish massage practitioners will ask about your general health and any current medication. You will lie on a special table or thick blanket, and the part of your body not being massaged will be kept warm under a towel. A light vegetable oil or talcum powder is usually used for lubrication. The massage techniques that they employ can be varied to make you feel more alert or to calm you down, according to your needs. Some practitioners have particular skills. For example, remedial massage aids healing of physical injury, manual lymph drainage aids expulsion of waste products through the lymphatic drainage system, which can enhance the immune system, and bio-dynamic massage aids release of psychological tensions, which can ease the symptoms of a number of allergic conditions, including asthma and irritable bowel syndrome.

CAUTIONS

Seek medical advice first if you have phlebitis, thrombosis, varicose veins, fever, severe back pain or a recently fractured bone. Avoid massage of the abdomen, legs and feet during the first three months of pregnancy. Also avoid massage if your skin is infected, bruised, or swollen. If you have cancer, you must consult a specially trained therapist. See also **Choosing a therapist**, p.139.

SELF-MASSAGE

Self-massage may not be as effective as having a massage from someone else, but it can bring similar benefits. Choose a vegetable oil, such as olive, almond or sunflower oil. If you have a sensitive skin, check that you do not react to the oil (see p.25). Add some **aromatherapy** oil if you wish (see p.150), choosing one that will stimulate or relax you, depending on your needs. Your room should be warm, and you should have a warm towel or robe handy.

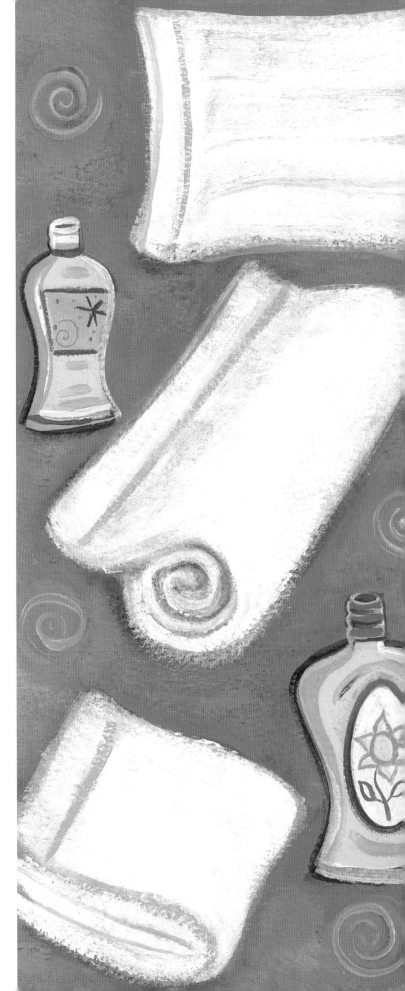

Start with your legs. Stroke them from your toes upwards, gradually making your touch firmer and kneading the muscles of your calves and the fronts of your thighs. Repeat the process on your arms and then stroke downwards on your neck. Then stand to massage your buttocks and lower back. Massage your upper back by briskly rubbing it with a towel. Then lie down and very gently massage your abdomen in a clockwise direction.

Finally, very gently massage your face, using small circular movements, starting at your chin and moving upwards. Stroke the skin of your forehead from the centre to the temples. Then wrap yourself in a warm towel or robe and rest for a while before having a warm shower or bath. If your intention with the massage was to induce a sense of calm, this is a good time to practise abdominal breathing and **muscle relaxation** (see p.124).

Aromatherapy

Aromatherapy oils are extracted from plants. They exert their effects after being absorbed into the body through the skin and mucous membranes of the nose. Eczema, rhinitis, asthma and irritable bowel syndrome can all benefit from aromatherapy, which also aids stress management.

Pure aromatherapy oils are both powerful and expensive. If they are to be applied to the skin or placed in a vaporizer, they are normally diluted in a 'carrier' oil, such as sweet almond oil or sunflower oil. A few drops of the essential oil itself, however, may be added to a bath. Your therapist will want to know about your medical history, especially about any skin problems, and about your lifestyle. Oils will be carefully chosen according to the desired effect, such as relaxation or stimulation. The therapist may give you a facial massage or a full body massage.

CAUTIONS

Ensure that your therapist is fully qualified, particularly if you are pregnant or have high blood pressure or epilepsy. Keep essential oils away from children and naked flames, and never take them by mouth, except under the supervision of a medically qualified therapist. See also **Choosing a therapist**, p.139.

SELF–HELP AROMATHERAPY

If you have a sensitive skin, it is important to test the carrier oil and the aromatherapy oil (see p.25) before applying them to large areas of skin. Do not apply near the eyes. Always dilute aromatherapy oils carefully, according to the manufacturer's instructions (except for lavender oil on burns and tea tree oil on insect stings). Use inhalations with care if you have asthma or are prone to nosebleeds. (See p.149 for **self-massage**.)

Peppermint: Use in low dilution to relieve spasm such as that experienced in IBS (see p.34) or as a nasal decongestant. Avoid taking homeopathic medicines at the same time, and do not use for children under the age of 12.

German camomile: Use for digestive disorders, insomnia and headaches. Its anti-inflammatory action may help to reduce allergies such as asthma and hay fever, and to soothe the skin, although it can cause a skin reaction in some people. Avoid during pregnancy, and test on your skin before use.

Lavender: Has a sedative and anti-spasmodic action. Use after insect stings, for nervous tension and digestive disorders.

Rosemary: Has a stimulant action and can relieve headache and digestive disorders. Avoid during pregnancy and if you have raised blood pressure or epilepsy.

Hypnotherapy

In hypnotherapy, the practitioner induces a trance-like state, rather like daydreaming, in which you are deeply relaxed and open to suggestion. Contrary to popular belief, you cannot be made to do anything that you do not wish to do. Hypnotherapy can relieve stress and is of value in allergic disorders, including IBS and food addictions, asthma, eczema and skin conditions. If you consult a practitioner, the treatment session usually lasts about an hour and may have to be repeated on a weekly basis.

CAUTIONS

Ensure that your practitioner is fully qualified and trustworthy. Hypnotherapy is not suitable if you have epilepsy. If you have a serious psychiatric disorder, such as severe depression or psychosis, consult your psychiatrist before embarking on any type of hypnotherapy. See also **Choosing a therapist**, p.139.

SELF-HYPNOSIS

Most people can learn how to induce self-hypnosis, either from a therapist, which is probably the best way, or from tapes and books. Regular daily practice for 20–30 minutes is helpful. You will need to find a warm place,

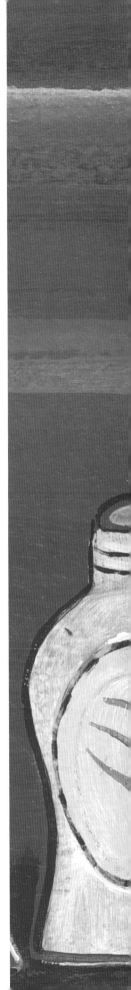

151

GETTING ADVICE

where you can adopt a comfortable position, and will not be disturbed.

Imagine yourself walking along a path, or down a long flight of stairs. Count backwards from ten to zero as your body relaxes. Then start repeating to yourself positive phrases that describe what you wish to achieve, such as 'Every day, and in every way, I am getting better and better'. Alternatively, you can make yourself an audiotape starting, perhaps, with music that you find soothing or natural sounds, such as waves on a beach or wind in trees. These can be followed by repetition of your phrase or phrases, so that you can listen and relax more effectively. When you are ready, imagine yourself walking back along the route you first chose, but this time count from zero to ten, as you bring yourself out of your hypnotic state.

Reflexology

Reflexologists believe that the different organs and parts of the body are represented, rather like a map, on special areas of the feet and hands. By massaging the feet and applying pressure to the areas that represent the different organs, reflexologists believe that they can stimulate the body to heal itself and overcome allergies such as asthma and eczema.

A reflexology session usually lasts about an hour, and at the first session the therapist will ask about your medical history and lifestyle. Reflexology can interfere with the action of any medication, so your reflexologist will want to know about what, if anything, you are taking and whether you are also consulting a herbalist, homeopath or aromatherapist. Lubricants are not used, as they would make the skin too slippery to apply pressure effectively. You may notice a 'healing crisis', such as a headache or tiredness, the following day.

CAUTIONS

It is important to check with your doctor if you have any long-term medical condition such as a thyroid disorder or diabetes. You should avoid having a reflexology treatment during the first three months of pregnancy. See also **Choosing a therapist**, p.139.

Shiatsu

Shiatsu has developed from traditional Chinese medicine, but includes some Western influences. The practitioner will take a detailed medical history, before applying pressure and massage to various areas of the body to stimulate the flow of energy within it, which enhances healing and a return to health. The treatment is robust, but should leave you feeling relaxed. You may develop a healing crisis afterwards, such as a headache or tiredness, but this is usually brief and energy levels are later improved. Shiatsu can be a particularly helpful way of relieving migraines.

CAUTIONS

Be sure to tell the practitioner if you are pregnant or have any chronic condition, such as AIDS, CFS, cancer, high blood pressure, epilepsy, osteoporosis, thrombosis or varicose veins, as some shiatsu techniques are unsuitable for these conditions. Eating, drinking alcohol, having a hot bath or shower, or taking strenuous exercise immediately before or after treatment may counteract its effect. See also **Choosing a therapist**, p.139.

Western herbalism

The remedies used in Western herbalism, which are derived from plants grown all over the world, both restore health and maintain it. The remedies are extracted from the leaves, flowers, roots and other parts of the plant as a mix of active ingredients, and herbalists believe that these act together to give a stronger effect, but one that is, at the same time, gentle. By contrast, the pharmaceutical industry takes great care to isolate the single ingredient in a plant that is most likely to produce the desired effect. This makes standardization easier and the medicine usually acts more quickly than if a herbal extract is used, but adverse side effects are more likely.

Plants contain complex chemicals, which can influence the chemical processes within the body and enable the immune system to act more effectively. The exact modes of action are not fully realized, but the powerful health-enhancing role of normal culinary plants is gradually being unravelled (see p.109). No doubt the plants that have been used for medicinal purposes will also, in time, become better understood.

The first consultation with a herbalist usually lasts about an hour, but follow-up appointments are generally shorter. The herbalist will ask about your current symptoms, medical history and lifestyle, and may also wish to examine you. Standards of training for herbal practitioners vary considerably in different parts of the world, as does legislation regarding which herbs can be sold.

CAUTIONS

Always keep your doctor and herbal practitioner fully informed about treatment that the other has prescribed. Consult your doctor before changing the dosage of your conventional medication.

If you notice any new symptoms or your allergic symptoms worsen, obtain advice promptly. Do not self-medicate with herbs if you are taking any regular prescribed medication, have heart disease, high blood pressure, glaucoma or are pregnant. Remember that plants can be difficult to identify and many are poisonous, so take great care if you gather your own herbs from the wild. See also **Choosing a therapist**, p.139.

Staying allergy-free

The dramatic rise in allergies and intolerances has been called 'the modern epidemic'. Hopefully, though, this book has shown you that if you suffer from allergies, it doesn't have to mean that you are doomed to ill-health. It is possible to overcome allergies and, in addition, by following the treatments or remedies suggested throughout this book, you can go on to enjoy an allergy-free life.

In order to maintain an allergy-free life, it is important to support your ongoing health and vitality generally and to make a few lifestyle changes.

- Eat healthily: remember to eat a wide range of different foods, balancing your intake of protein, carbohydrate and fat, and to drink plenty of water.
- Consider supplements: boost your nutrient levels by taking vitamins and mineral supplements and treat specific conditions with herbal remedies.
- Exercise regularly: try yoga or tai chi, for example, and learn to manage your stress.
- Create a lo-allergy environment
- Treat specific symptoms or ailments: look at all the available therapies and chose the right one for you.

For many of us, allergies can prove to be a wake-up call, nudging us to listen to our bodies and to look after them. Make the most of this opportunity!

Further reading

Allergy Elimination Diet, The, Jill Carter and Alison Edwards (Vermilion)

Allergy Free Cookbook, The, Michelle Berriedale-Johnson (Thorsons)

Allergy Free Eating, Liz Reno and Joanna Devrais (Celestial Arts)

Allergy Sourcebook, The, Merla Zellerbach (Lowell House)

Alternative Answers to Asthma and Allergies, Barbara Rowlands and Alan Watkins (Marshall Publishing)

Arthritis, Allergy, Nutrition and the Environment, John Mansfield (Thorsons)

Chemical Children, Peter Mansfield and Jean Monro (Century Paperbacks)

Complete Guide to Food Allergy and Intolerance, The, Jonathan Brostoff and Linda Gamlin (Bloomsbury)

Complete Guide to Integrated Medicine, David Peters and Anne Woodham (Dorling Kindersley)

Could it be an Allergy?, Joe Fitzgibbon (Newleaf)

Environmental Medicine in Clinical Practice, Honor Anthony, Keith Eaton and Jonathan Maberly (BSAENM Publications)

Everyday Wheat-free and Gluten-free Cookbook, The, Michelle Berriedale-Johnson (Grub Street)

Planning for a Healthy Baby, Belinda Barnes and Suzanne Gail Bradley (Ebury Press)

Textbook of Natural Medicine, Joseph E. Pizzorno and Michael T. Murray (eds) (Churchill Livingstone)

Vitamin Alphabet, The, Christina Scott-Moncrieff (Collins and Brown)

Your Home, Your Health and Well-Being, David Rousseau, W.J. Rea and Jean Enwright (Ten Speed Press)

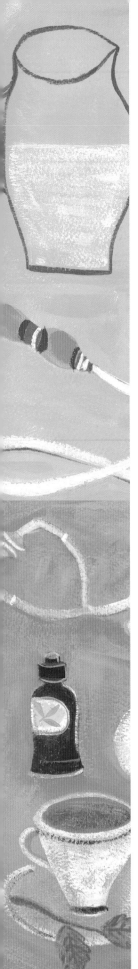

Useful addresses

SOCIETIES AND ASSOCIATIONS

British Society for Allergy, Environmental and Nutritional Medicine
PO Box 7
Powys, Knighton LD7 1WF
UK
Tel: (01547) 550380 / Fax: (01547) 550339

American Academy of Environmental Medicine
7701 East Kellogg Suite 625
Wichita, Kansas 67207
USA
Tel: (316) 684 5500 / Fax: (316) 684 5709

Canadian Society for Clinical Ecology and Environmental Medicine
479 Roncesvalles Avenue
Toronto
Ontario M6R 2N4
CANADA
Tel: (416) 536 9903

Australasian College of Nutritional and Environmental Medicine
13 Hilton Street
Beaumaris
Victoria 3193
AUSTRALIA
Tel: (395) 896088 / Fax: (395) 895158
Email: acnem@mail.austasia.net

HOMEOPATHY

British Homeopathic Association
15 Clerkenwell Close
London EC1R 0AA
UK
Tel: (020) 7566 7800 / Fax: (020) 7566 7815

National Center for Homeopathy
801 North Fairfax Street, Suite 306
Alexandria
Virginia 22314
USA
Tel: (703) 548 7790 / Fax: (703) 548 7792

PRODUCTS BY POST (This list does not imply endorsement of any company or product)

Allergy Care (for foods)
Pollard's Yard
Wood Street
Taunton TA1 1UP
UK
Tel: (01823) 325022 or (01823) 325023

American Health and Nutrition Inc. (for foods)
3990 Varsity Drive
Ann Arbor
Michigan 48108
USA
Tel: (734) 677 5570 / Fax: (734) 677 5572
Email: ahn@organictrading.com

Allergy Aid Centre (for foods and cleaning products)
325 Chapel Street
Prahran
Victoria 3181
AUSTRALIA
Tel: (395) 297348 / Fax: (395) 298459

Index